# DEVELOPING YOUR COMPASSION STRENGTHS

This practical book suggests ways in which healthcare students and practitioners can develop their compassion strengths.

Discussing what compassion is and means, it includes a new compassion strength model and a series of exercises the reader can use for reflecting on and developing their practice. A hallmark of healthcare practice is compassion, yet there is a lack of understanding as to what compassion is and how it can be developed in practice. The book begins with the challenge of defining compassion, particularly looking at healthcare contexts and making links between self-care and caring for others. It then presents a new, evidence-based holistic model that brings together key elements of compassion for self and other, along with a scale that readers can measure themselves against. Identifying eight strengths "self-care, connection, communication, competency, empathy, interpersonal skills, character, and engagement" Durkin provides the theoretical background to each, accompanied with suggestions for practice and reflective activities. It ends with a selection of vignettes that readers can use to try out their strengths.

Highlighting the concept of compassion strengths, and compassion as a way of being, this is an essential read for healthcare students and practitioners, whether involved in direct patient care or management.

**Mark Durkin** is a lecturer in Psychology at Leeds Trinity University, UK.

# DEVELOPING YOUR COMPASSION STRENGTHS

## A Guide for Healthcare Students and Practitioners

*Mark Durkin*

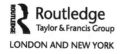
Routledge
Taylor & Francis Group

LONDON AND NEW YORK

Designed cover image: © Getty Images

First published 2023
by Routledge
4 Park Square, Milton Park, Abingdon, Oxon OX14 4RN

and by Routledge
605 Third Avenue, New York, NY 10158

*Routledge is an imprint of the Taylor & Francis Group, an informa business*

*British Library Cataloguing-in-Publication Data*
A catalogue record for this book is available from the British Library

ISBN: 978-1-032-23245-4 (hbk)
ISBN: 978-1-032-23208-9 (pbk)
ISBN: 978-1-003-27642-5 (ebk)

DOI: 10.4324/9781003276425

Typeset in Bembo
by MPS Limited, Dehradun

*To my son Callum, my mum Maureen, and my granddaughter Emilia Rae Durkin for their compassion and strength always.*

# CONTENTS

# FIGURES

# TABLES

# BOXES

# FOREWORD

"When you wake up in the morning, tell yourself: the people I deal with today will be meddling, ungrateful, arrogant, dishonest, jealous and surly. They are like this because they can't tell good from evil. But I have seen the beauty of good, and the ugliness of evil, and have recognized that the wrongdoer has a nature related to my own - not of the same blood and birth, but the same mind, and possessing a share of the divine. And so, none of them can hurt me. No one can implicate me in ugliness. Nor can I feel angry at my relative or hate him. We were born to work together like feet, hands and eyes, like the two rows of teeth, upper and lower. To obstruct each other is unnatural. To feel anger at someone, to turn your back on him: these are unnatural."

*Marcus Aurelius*

It is a pleasure to introduce this excellent new book on compassion strengths. I'll leave it to the author to explain how compassion relates to deep philosophical perspectives and key research areas across psychology – he does so better than I could here. Rather, I'd like to note how this book fits within an emerging tradition within psychology, which highlights why this book is timely and needed.

Prior to the 1950s psychology had the dual aim of combatting mental distress and promoting character excellence (Alex et al., 2006). In the aftermath of the World Wars this holistic focus became lost, with the focus of the discipline being shaped by the urgent need to treat trauma, as well as understanding the social psychology of how and why people were capable of committing such atrocities. The development of the United States Department of Veteran Affairs (1989) and the National Institute of Mental Health (1949) (which exclusively focused on *ill-*health) funded valuable research into such topics as the neurology of brain trauma, treatment of post-traumatic illness, and social conformity and authoritarianism. Whilst this research (and the associated funding) was most welcome, an intended consequence was to shape psychology away from positive characteristics towards an over-focus on the negative in life. As Abraham Maslow warned as early as 1954.

> The science of psychology has been far more successful on the negative than on the positive side; it has revealed to us much about man's shortcomings, his illnesses, his sins, but little about his potentialities, his virtues, his achievable aspirations, or his psychological height. It is as if psychology had voluntarily restricted itself to only half its rightful jurisdiction, and that the darker, meaner half.

The study of self-compassion and compassion thus became marginalized, despite having been considered essential to life by philosophical and religious perspectives – and, indeed, by people in their own lives. This epitomizes the problems of psychology overfocusing on the negative in life; such a focus prevents psychology from addressing many key questions about life and being able to speak to many issues of importance to individuals. Such was the case at the end of the 20th Century, where it was difficult for research into topics such as compassion to be taken seriously as a mainstream part of psychology.

The positive psychology movement emerged in the early 2000s, promoted by Martin Seligman, the President of the American Psychological Association (APA) as his key executive initiative. "Movement" perhaps overstates the case, as positive psychology was adopted by researchers and practitioners for differing reasons and with different objectives. Early on we highlighted that the movement could go in two directions; towards integration with "negative" psychology or becoming a separate area of inquiry that focus exclusively on the "positive", entrenching the split in the discipline (Wood et al., 2021). Sadly, the latter perspective largely dominated (Linley et al., 2009). In 2010 we aimed to promote a more holistic discipline, with "positive clinical psychology", which aimed to equally focus on an intervene on both the "positive" and "negative" in life. There are several reasons why this is needed. First, well-being normally exists on a continuum from positive to negative such that the two cannot be meaningfully separated (Wood & Tarrier, 2010). Anxiety is continuous with calmness, depression with "happiness" (Siddayway et al., 2017). Further, we find that the benefits of moving from, say, anxiety to calmness continue across the whole continuum, and don't just stop when we reach the mid-point of neither anxious nor calm. This understanding is represented across this book, through a focus on both fostering the positive rather than being satisfied with addressing the negative. Second, positive characteristics are often stronger predictors of well-being than negative ones, as seen by our work into gratitude, a concept that is well represented throughout the chapters. Third, positive characteristics confer resilience, where the strengths we develop help us cope with challenging life events when they occur for us (Johnson et al., 2010a&b). The fostering of such resilience through developing the strength of compassion is a key aim of this book. Indeed, the book fundamentally fits within our work showing that the use of psychological strengths leads to improved well-being over time (Wood et al., 2011). Third, interventions that improve the positive in life are often as effective in treating dysfunction as those which specifically focus on the dysfunction itself (Geraghty et al., 2010a&b).

The opening quote is from Stoic philosopher Markus Aurelius, the scholar and Emperor of Rome. This is one of my favourite quotes, in part due to how it contrasts with the "just think positively" type of self-help book. Far from suggesting that we start our days with positive thoughts, Aurelius encourages us to think about the negative interactions that we have during the day; the meddling, ungrateful, arrogant, dishonest, jealous, and surly people that we will meet (and I can think of a few people who manage to have each characteristic simultaneously). And yet the advice is intensive positive, as the focus is on pre-empting these interactions with such a mind-set that will enable us to react to negative social interactions with compassion. Aurelius reminds us that such negative social behaviours emerge from a poor understanding of the nuances of life that lead us to behave in a positive, pro-social manner that enhances our well-being and the well-being of others. He encourages us to keep in mind our shared humanity, and that others cannot directly hurt us, but rather hurt emerges from our own reactions – and these reactions we can control. Like it or not, every day we *will* meet people who are meddling, ungrateful or otherwise unskilled in their behaviour. Pretending otherwise will not prevent these interactions. We could choose to just be reactive to the situation, and likely wind ourselves up considerably, being authors of our own suffering. Or, alternatively, we could mentally prepare ourselves to react with compassion. However, deciding to react with compassions is one thing, actually doing so is quite another. It takes hard work to train ourselves to behave with compassion in difficult situations, which are exactly the kind of situations where we most need it. Like Aurelius and the rest of the Stoics, they can be considered ahead of their time as the first wellbeing practitioners. In fact, their teachings still resonate today. Whether you are a coach, psychologist, nurse or other healthcare practitioner the compassion strengths presented in this book are and should be as very much a part of your training as learning about the clinical skills needed for your work. We need to develop knowledge and understanding of compassion and self-compassion and why it is needed. We need to practice the discipline and understand the fundamental aspects needed to enable us to act compassionately when in the heat of the moment. This is of paramount importance for every student and practitioner working in healthcare where compassion is key to ensuring that patients and clients receive not just the best clinical care but the compassionate too. Fortunately, we have this book to guide us through this process.

Professor Alex M. Wood
Leeds Trinity University

# ACKNOWLEDGEMENTS

I am extremely grateful to all the staff, students and service users who shared their valuable knowledge and experience with me to help develop the ideas within this book.

Thank you to my good friends and family close and far who have always supported me no matter what. My mother and Malc deserve a special thanks for always being there for me with encouragement, love, food, and supportive words. Also, my amazing son Callum, daughter in law Megan, granddaughter Emilia, and dogs. Thank you for being there, being you and making me a very proud father and grandfather. To my partner Sian, Eva, Noah, the dogs, and extended family, I am always extremely grateful for your love and support. A massive thanks to Professor Jerome Carson for recommending I write this book, for reviewing earlier versions, and your guidance, counsel and many years of encouragement over the years. Thank you to those who have offered their views and opinions and helped me format pages and the book cover. I would like to extend a big thank you to my good friend Carl Simms for his assistance with the image for the book. An extra special thank you to Grace McInnes and Evie Lonsdale at Routledge for their constant advice and guidance throughout the writing process. Thank you to Professors Russell and Dawne Gurbutt for their thoughts on earlier versions of this book.

# 1

# INTRODUCTION TO THE BOOK

---

**MEASURE**

In this chapter you can measure your compassion strengths and help identify what your greatest strengths are and what areas you can work on.

---

## Introduction

This book is about compassion, compassion strengths to be exact. While most books will look at self-compassion, or how organisations can foster compassion, this book's primary focus is on practitioners and how they can develop their compassion strengths. Most blame the lack of compassion on organisations rather than the practitioners themselves. This book is different, however, as it places the responsibility for compassion at the feet of the very people who work in these environments. That is not to say that these places of work do not have their barriers to compassionate care, but that students and practitioners can develop their knowledge and skills associated with each strength and learn how to demonstrate them in practice. They may be the most compassionate person in the world, but as one student said to me until you have been into practice you never really know how to do it and how hard it is with actual patients.

Organisations are made up of individuals too, so they are collectively responsible for compassion. To this end, there is a section in the last chapter that explores how organisations can help promote compassion strengths. Specifically, this book focuses on the actions of compassion in healthcare and introduces the reader to a set of eight compassion strengths. A series of exercises can be found in the last chapter to help you, your colleagues and the wider healthcare organisation develop compassion strengths further.

DOI: 10.4324/9781003276425-1

## Why a book about compassion strengths?

Why is this book necessary, why do students and practitioners need another book about compassion? There are a plethora of books, articles, and workshops about developing compassion. Most training programmes for healthcare students and practitioners offer some kind of course for learning about compassion too. This goes to show just how important learning about compassion is for students and practitioners, even more so for patient outcomes. Each author or programme provider will have something unique to offer in their understanding of compassion and in many respects, this book is my contribution to the ever-growing literature and knowledge about compassion.

This book is influenced not only by my research, and experience but by my journey with compassion. In April 2016, I realised a goal of mine when I got the opportunity to give a TEDx talk at the University of Bolton. From my early days as a mature student, like most, I became obsessed with watching TED talks and digesting all the fascinating information from the great presenters that have stood in the red circle. I remember thinking, one day it might be me up there, but it would be a long time in the future. Maybe if I became a professor and had something interesting to share. Little did I know I would get my chance sooner than that. At the time, I was a master's student and had just started to research self-compassion and compassion for others among healthcare students and did not have a clue what to give my talk on. I have always found both remarkably interesting but the more I learned about them, the more I realised how they applied to my life at various stages. It eventually became clear that this was what my talk must be about. I gave the talk, called Agents of Compassion. In it, I named five agents of compassion that could be demonstrated to self and others based on the experiences I have had with people during some tough times in my life. The five agents of compassion are awareness, wiser judgements, communication courage, and patience. You can watch the talk here https://youtu.be/AViAAAhwMsk

As I went on to study for my Ph.D., I started to wonder if the things I had spoken about in my talk could be found among healthcare staff, in particular nurses. This then became the focus of my research. What influences me, is the sheer power of compassion, and how it can transform people, both the giver and receiver. For me, it is seen most in healthcare settings because this is when we need it most, in our times of heartache and suffering. It takes courage and strength to face distress head-on and support someone in their time of need. Therefore, I chose to focus on developing compassion as a strength in healthcare. However, compassion is a human condition and I hope that what I present in this book can translate far beyond practice and into all our lives.

## Problems/challenges with compassion in healthcare settings

Compassion is at the heart of care, and it is what patients need most when being cared for at the most vulnerable moments in their lives. It is written into most policies, and constitutions, and is a key feature of ethical codes for practitioners in healthcare institutions across the globe. In the UK, America, New Zealand, Australia, and Canada, Compassion is considered a necessity. The National Health Service Constitution (2015) consists of a set of values that underpin the work that the NHS does with each of the individual organisations able to tailor these values to their own needs. Compassion is one of these values and is said as being *"central to the care we provide and respond with humanity and kindness to each person's pain, distress, anxiety, or need"* (NHS Constitution, 2015, p.5). Yet, despite its importance, there is evidence both anecdotal and from reports in healthcare that something is missing with compassion. Reports in the UK such as the Francis report (2013) point to a culture of poor care underpinned by a lack of compassion towards patients. Despite several positive accounts from patients and their relatives, these reports show that many had been left to suffer unnecessarily from a lack of compassion and that these stories of neglect were due to staff shortages, and the organisation losing sight of its goal to provide safe standards of care. This problem is also not just limited to the UK. In America, equivalent results have been found, with more than half of patients reporting feeling that their practitioner did not treat them with compassion (Lown, 2011).

Sometimes this is because the definition of compassion and what it means in practice is not clear. Other reasons include feeling overwhelmed and short-staffed for why practitioners struggle to provide compassionate care (Papadopoulos et al., 2016). Although practitioners are dedicated to showing compassion, issues of poor care have raised concerns about the current state of compassion in healthcare organisations around the world. Healthcare professionals struggle to distinguish between compassion and similar terms such as empathy, while others find their working environment reduces their capacity to be compassionate (Sinclair et al., 2016a). Others suggest that there is a blame culture in healthcare where practitioners place the blame for their lack of compassion at the foot of the government or policymakers with excuses of short staff, stress, and a litany of other reasons (Richards & Borglin, 2019). In response to this, a change in thinking is needed from one of blame to mature responsibility where staff and organisations take the steps to enable compassion to flourish.

## Compassion education

Traditionally, so-called "soft skills" such as compassion would have taken a back seat in healthcare education training to the biological model which is more concerned with explaining disease and illness in medical terminology. This view typically places less emphasis on psycho-social wellbeing (Draper & Louw, 2007). This can also lead to detachment from the human aspect of patient care. Compassion helps forge the connections between practitioner and patient. However, despite this, there are very few educational programmes for compassion in healthcare. Most work on a limited definition and one-dimensional view of compassion. Despite its importance across all of healthcare, compassion also tends to be embedded into other curricula such as end-of-life care, caring conversations, or be focused on leadership (Sinclair et al., 2021). The most effective courses teach about compassion through a blend of patient narratives, self-care, reflective writing, clinical exposure, scenario-based learning, communication, and role modelling (Menezes et al., 2021). Programmes for developing a compassionate mind in therapy students can help them become more self-compassionate (Beaumont et al., 2016a,b,c). Very few, if any, try to teach the fundamentals of compassion. My research shows that teaching compassion strengths can help nursing students develop their compassion and apply it to their work (Durkin et al., 2022). Although this was with nursing students, the compassion strengths model applies to other helping professions. When standards suggest it is a trait that all practitioners should aspire to, compassion becomes a desirable rather than an essential element of their training. More is needed to make the behaviour of compassion explicit. This is the aim of this book.

## Who is this book for?

This book is for healthcare students and practitioners, nurses, psychologists, physicians, social workers, therapists, and anyone who works in a healthcare setting and cares for other people.

## How will it help you?

The background information presented in this book will give you more insight and understanding of compassion, while the chapters on compassion strengths will give you the information and things to consider when developing these strengths. The exercises in the last chapter will help you improve and sustain your compassion strengths. The scale will help you measure your compassion strengths as and when you believe it fit. However, because things outside of our control can reduce your strengths, I would recommend measuring yourself at regular intervals to track your progress over time. This can also help you see what affects your compassion strengths.

## Measuring compassion

Can compassion be measured? This is a key question in healthcare. Also, should students and practitioners be assessed for compassion? What do you think?

_____

_____

_____

_____

_____

Not only do I believe that it can be measured, but I also think that it should be, and healthcare staff assessed for it in the same way they would for any other skill of strength. Assessment promotes understanding, while feedback helps us see what can be done to improve care and helps educators make judgements about staff needs and course acceptance and progression for students. Assessing staff and students for their strengths of compassion, can help recognise needs, promote learning, and improve patient outcomes. By not assessing for compassion organisations run the risk of communicating to staff and students that it is not valued in practice (Wright et al., 2019).

So, before we go any further, use this section of the book to explore your compassion strengths using the Bolton Compassion Strengths Indicators scale. This will help you to see where your compassion strengths lie and give you a platform for developing them further using the exercises in this book.

## The Bolton Compassion Strengths Indicators

The Bolton Compassion Strengths Indicators (Durkin et al., 2021) is a 48-item measure of compassion strengths. It is based on extensive research into the characteristics of compassion. While it is recommended to be used as a single measure of overall compassion, each strength can be measured individually. It can help you to think of the scale as your learner's needs assessment, where you can name your strongest areas of compassion and what you might need to develop further. Reflect on your experience and understanding of the following statements below. Rate them using the 1–6 scale for whether you agree with each one

1.  = Definitely not like me
2.  = Generally, not like me
3.  = Slightly not like me
4.  = Slightly like me
5.  = Generally, like me
6.  = Definitely like me

The purpose of this scale is to help you name and develop your compassionate strengths. Please read the following set of statements carefully. They have purposefully been left blank in certain statements so that you can fill them out with your profession. Using the scoring guide score each statement with the number that honestly reflects your experience as a student or practitioner. Please make sure that you answer all the statements. Fill in the blank sections with your profession and the appropriate terminology for the people you care for (Client/Patient/Service User).

**TABLE 1.1** The Bolton Compassion Strengths Indicators

| | |
|---|---|
| 1. I evaluate care effectively | |
| 2. I encourage caregivers to be supportive | |
| 3. I am aware of whether or not a _____ interpretation of something is the same as mine | |
| 4. I am gentle in my approach to _____ | |

(*Continued*)

**TABLE 1.1** (*Continued*)

| | |
|---|---|
| 5. I explain symptoms and what they mean to help alleviate any worries _____ may have | |
| 6. Honesty is an important quality for a _____ to have | |
| 7. I try to be as open as possible with _____ | |
| 8. I develop a shared decision when making a treatment plan | |
| 9. I like to make small talk with _____ at every opportunity | |
| 10. I often take time out to ask _____ about the state of their health | |
| 11. I listen to the complete message before making a judgement about the speaker | |
| 12. Listening helps me understand the speaker's intentions | |
| 13. Where appropriate, I adapt my _____ practice to meet unpredictable circumstances | |
| 14. I stick to my promises when I agree to help _____ | |
| 15. I believe in myself no matter what | |
| 16. I carry out an effective discharge plan | |
| 17. I feel in control of my life | |
| 18. When _____ start talking, I do not interrupt them | |
| 19. I find people to be the most interesting thing in life | |
| 20. When I am feeling burned out, I soothe myself with comforting words | |
| 21. I prepare _____ appropriately for diagnostic procedures | |
| 22. Working with _____ energises me | |
| 23. The ability to imagine myself in another's situation contributes to providing quality healthcare | |
| 24. I enjoy speaking to _____ and finding out how they are doing | |
| 25. Respecting the _____ is just as important as the care they receive | |
| 26. _____ would describe me as showing warmth | |
| 27. I am confident about the future | |

(*Continued*)

**TABLE 1.1** (*Continued*)

| | |
|---|---|
| 28. I believe that empathy is important for the therapeutic relationship between _____ and patient/client | |
| 29. My ability to understand how _____ and their families are feeling helps me care for them | |
| 30. Trust is an important part of the caring relationship | |
| 31. I am able to accurately assess the effectiveness of preventative health advice to meet the _____ needs | |
| 32. I can make my _____ feel better when I understand their feelings | |
| 33. Despite the challenges I gain pleasure from caring for _____ | |
| 34. I have respect for my _____ needs | |
| 35. I provide relevant and current health information to _____ in a way that they understand, and which gives them the option to choose | |
| 36. I feel I am approachable to _____ | |
| 37. I believe that the ability to view things from the _____ perspective can lead to better care | |
| 38. I listen to what others have to say when they are talking | |
| 39. My life experiences have prepared me to deal with whatever comes my way | |
| 40. When there are no clear solutions to my problems sometimes fate or God can help | |
| 41. I take time out to listen to _____ concerns | |
| 42. I think that the best way to take care of a _____ is to try and understand what they are going through | |
| 43. I do not see each _____ as a whole person | |
| 44. I ask _____ to discuss any matters about their stay in hospital | |
| 45. I feel a sense of joy from meeting new people and finding out more about them | |
| 46. Being a _____ serves a greater purpose | |
| 47. I pay close attention to what my _____ are saying | |
| 48. I ask _____ if they have any problems following what has been recommended | |

## Scoring the BCSI

Individual compassion strength scores are computed by adding the responses for each item. A total compassion strengths score is achieved by adding the total score from each strength together. Please note that item 43 is reversed scored.

This gives you a sign of what your overall strengths are. Higher scores on each signify a higher score for that strength and overall compassion strengths when combined. Do not worry if they are low as this can help you understand what areas you need to work on or that other factors such as work might be affecting your strengths. Even if you have high scores across all strengths, you can still use the book to develop your compassion strengths further with a compassionate understanding.

## What your scores mean for overall compassion strengths

A score of 240 or above means you have high overall compassion strengths. This suggests that you are strong in all eight strengths and show them often in your work. Things change over time, so it is always recommended that you continue to measure yourself and do the work to keep your compassion strengths.

A score of between 145 and 239 means you have a moderate amount of compassion strengths and there are strengths you need to develop further. You might be stronger with certain strengths such as communication but not with others, such as self-care. Looking at your scores for each strength will help you find which areas need your attention right now.

A score of 144 and below suggests that your compassion strengths need to be improved. This is because you are a student and have little experience with compassion. You might be feeling burned out and not very compassionate. Whatever the reason, this is a good sign that you need to build your compassion strengths.

## What your scores mean for each compassion strength

A score of 18 or less shows that you need to work on this compassion strength. You might struggle with this compassion strength, or it may be that you have not learned enough about it.

A score of 19–29 suggests that you might want to reflect on your strengths and explore ways to make this compassion stronger. This would show that you have insight into this strength but may not have used it as much as you could.

A score of 30 and above shows that this is a strong compassion strength for you. This compassion strength is one that you do very well in. However, as with any strength you need to continue working on it.

Report your scores in the table below to get a sign of where your compassion strengths lie on the range of scores.

**TABLE 1.2** Scoring key for the BCSIs

|  | SC | EM | CH | CON | COM | COMP | INT | ENG | Total |
|---|---|---|---|---|---|---|---|---|---|
| High |  |  |  |  |  |  |  |  |  |
| Moderate |  |  |  |  |  |  |  |  |  |
| Low |  |  |  |  |  |  |  |  |  |

What are your strongest compassion strengths?

_____
_____
_____
_____
_____

Do you agree with them?

_____
_____
_____
_____
_____

What compassion strengths do you need to work on?

_____
_____
_____
_____
_____

Do you agree with them?

_____
_____
_____
_____
_____

In measuring your compassion strengths, you have just completed the first section of the META model. But what is the META model?

## The META model

In addition to the compassion strengths model, this book includes a model of learning and behaviour change called META The dictionary definition of META means to: involve change, metamorphose (to change into something), outside the

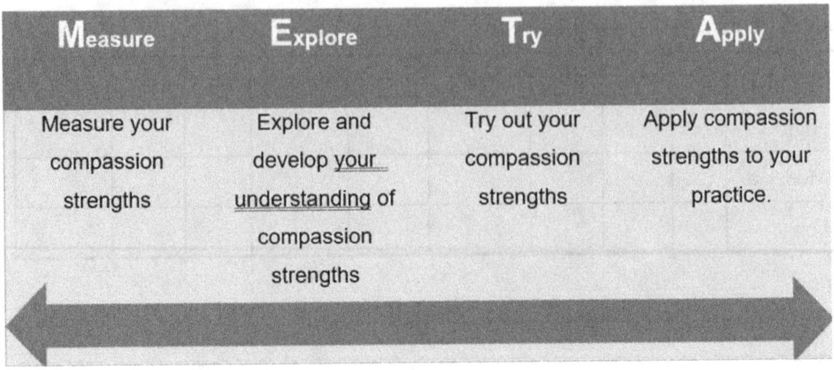

| Measure | Explore | Try | Apply |
|---------|---------|-----|-------|
| Measure your compassion strengths | Explore and develop your understanding of compassion strengths | Try out your compassion strengths | Apply compassion strengths to your practice. |

**FIGURE 1.1** The META model

normal limits of something, change, occurring later, and transcending (Cambridge Online Dictionary, 2018; Merriam-Webster Online Dictionary, 2018). Where in this book META is an acronym, the significance of these definitions is relevant to the underlying meaning behind the model. It is about change, growth, and development. The overall aim of the META model is to guide the development of compassion strengths, through the measure, exploration, testing, and application of skills learned within the compassion strengths model.

The Bolton Compassion Strengths Indicators, in this chapter is the **Measure** element. Chapters 3 to 13 allow you to **Explore** the background of compassion, compassion in healthcare settings, the compassion strengths, while Chapter 14 has in it exercises that you can use to **Try** out and develop your compassion strengths. For the final part of the model, there are examples of how you can **Apply** what you have learned to your practice.

## How META features in this book

**TABLE 1.3** How META features in this book

| Measure | Explore | Try | Apply |
|---------|---------|-----|-------|
| In the first chapter, you will be invited to measure your compassion strengths. | In Chapters 2 to 13, you will be able to explore the background of compassion and the compassion strengths model. You can explore each strength in detail too. | In the closing chapter, you will have the opportunity to try out the exercises that will help you build your strengths. | In the concluding chapter, you will see how compassion strengths can be applied to your practice. |

## How to use this book

This book has been designed with you in mind. It aims to share insightful information about compassion in healthcare, what compassion means, and how it is considered from various points of view. It also includes exercises that will help you develop your compassion strengths through a range of activities and exercises. This book also features theory and useful examples from positive psychology that can help you understand your psychology, build resilience and improve wellbeing.

You can choose how you work through the book too. You might want to focus on certain compassion strengths first, especially those that you feel you might need to explore in more detail. Equally, you could go through the book chapter by chapter. With the exercises, you also have the choice to c pick or try one at a time. It is entirely up to you. My advice would be to work through each one at a time. They have been developed and each chapter was created to follow on from the earlier compassion strength to show how each combine and works together.

## Simple exercises

In each of the strength's chapters, you will find a quick and simple exercise that you can do to help you develop that compassion strength. These are meant to be as straight forward as possible so that you practice them in the moment without them taking up too much of your time. They have been adapted and developed based on evidenced research and practice in self-compassion and positive psychology.

## How often should you use the book?

I would suggest using the book each day. Going through the chapters and learning about each of the compassion strengths, and their indicators. This way you build up your strengths and can try them out in practice, all the time reflecting and learning new things about how you can apply them to your work. The amount of time you devote to the exercise in this book is entirely up to you. You have the conscious choice and free will. What I do know from research in positive psychology on GRIT, is that you must be self-disciplined and persistent. So, practice, practice, practice, as the more you put into it, the more you will get out.

## Journaling (reflective practice)

You will be expected to reflect on a lot of things throughout this book so it would be extremely helpful for you to journal about your experiences. At the end of each chapter, there is a question that asks you what you have learned that you did not know before. This can encourage learning, free up mental space, and give insight into personal thoughts and behaviours. You can use a book, or your laptop/ computer, it does not matter; it is about finding what works best for you.

## Work with others using this book

While the exercises can be done alone, they can also be done with others. Collaborating with a colleague or fellow student, even a student group, can help you get more out of the book as you work together to develop your compassion strengths and support each other's development. Hold meetings and see how these compassion strengths can be applied to your workplace.

## How this book is set out

### Chapter 1: Introduction

This chapter gives an overview of the book and the rationale for why it is needed and introduces the reader to the META model. It also includes the Bolton Compassion Strengths Indicators that practitioners can use to measure themselves for compassion strengths.

### Chapter 2: What is compassion

This chapter is about the background of compassion, its definition, and what that means. It also covers the different terms that are like compassion and distinguishes them from each other.

### Chapter 3: Compassion in healthcare

In Chapter 3 the focus is on compassion in healthcare settings. It explores the barriers and enablers to compassion in a practice setting.

### Chapter 4: Compassion strengths

In this chapter, we will look at the compassion strengths model and how each of the strengths applies to different healthcare professions.

### Chapter 5 to 12: Each of the compassion strengths

In these eight chapters, each one of the compassion strengths will be explored in detail. You will be able to reflect on each type and think of ways you can implement them into your practice. Over the next eight chapters, you will be introduced to each strength in more detail. Each chapter is set so that you can focus on one strength at a time. You can pick the ones that appeal to you most, or that you feel you could benefit most from. Each chapter follows a similar format covering, what it is, The opposite, The barriers, The benefits, The types, and Combing strengths.

### Chapter 13: Applications of compassion strengths

The concluding chapter will cover the diverse ways that compassion strengths can be applied to practice. It will also include exercises to help you develop your compassion strengths.

## Conclusion

Now we have reached the end of the first chapter, you should know what your compassion strengths are and what to expect from this book. You have been introduced to the META model and how it will guide you through each stage of the book as you explore the different compassion strengths. Before we get to the compassion strengths model and each strength, the book will investigate the background to compassion. The following chapters all have information about compassion and healthcare and will provide you with insight and knowledge so you can become more aware of compassion, and how to bring it into your practice. But first, in the next chapter, we will explore what compassion is.

## References

Beaumont, E., Durkin, M., Martin, C. J. H., & Carson, J. (2016a). Compassion for others, self-compassion, quality of life and mental well-being measures and their association with compassion fatigue and burnout in student midwives: A quantitative survey. *Midwifery*, *34*, 239–244.

Beaumont, E., Durkin, M., Hollins Martin, C. J., & Carson, J. (2016b). Measuring relationships between self-compassion, compassion fatigue, burnout and well-being in student counsellors and student cognitive behavioural psychotherapists: a quantitative survey. *Counselling and Psychotherapy Research*, *16*(1), 15–23.

Beaumont, E., Durkin, M., McAndrew, S., & Martin, C. R. (2016c). Using compassion focused therapy as an adjunct to trauma-focused CBT for fire service personnel suffering with trauma-related symptoms. *The Cognitive Behaviour Therapist*, *9*.E34

Draper, C., & Louw, G. (2007). What is medicine and what is a doctor? Medical students' perceptions and expectations of their academic and professional career. *Medical Teacher*, *29*(5), e100–e107.

Durkin, J., Jackson, D., & Usher, K. (2021). The expression and receipt of compassion through touch in a health setting; a qualitative study. *Journal of Advanced Nursing*, *77*(4), 1980–1991.

Durkin, M., Gurbutt, R., & Carson, J. (2022). Effectiveness of an online short compassion strengths course on nursing students compassion: A mixed methods non-randomised pilot study. *Nurse Education Today*, *111*, 105315.

Francis, R. (2013). *Report of the Mid Staffordshire NHS Foundation Trust: Public inquiry*. London: The Stationery Office (TSO).

Lown, B. A., Rosen, J., & Marttila, J. (2011). An agenda for improving compassionate care: A survey shows about half of patients say such care is missing. *Health Affairs*, *30*, 1772–1778.

Menezes, M. P., Guraya, S. Y., & Guraya, S. S. (2021). A systematic review of educational interventions and their impact on empathy and compassion of undergraduate medical students. *Frontiers in Medicine*, *2129*, 1–16.

Papadopoulos, I., Shea, S., Taylor, G., Pezzella, A., & Foley, L. (2016). Developing tools to promote culturally competent compassion, courage, and intercultural communication in healthcare. *Journal of Compassionate Health Care*, *3*(1), 2.

Richards, D. A., & Borglin, G. (2019). 'Shitty nursing' – The new normal?. *International Journal of Nursing Studies*, *91*, 148–152.

Sinclair, S., Kondejewski, J., Jaggi, P., Dennett, L., des Ordons, A. L. R., & Hack, T. F. (2021). What is the state of compassion education? A systematic review of compassion training in health care. *Academic Medicine*, *96*(7), 1057.

Sinclair, S., Norris, J. M., McConnell, S. J., Chochinov, H. M., Hack, T. F., Hagen, N. A., ... & Bouchal, S. R. (2016a). Compassion: A scoping review of the healthcare literature. *BMC Palliative Care*, *15*, 193–203. 10.1186/s12904-016-0080-0

The NHS Constitution: The NHS belongs to us all. (2015). London: Department of Health.

Wright, S. R., Boyd, V. A., & Ginsburg, S. (2019). The Hidden Curriculum of Compassionate Care: Can Assessment Drive Compassion? *Academic medicine: Journal of the Association of American Medical Colleges*, 94, 1164–1169.

# 2

# UNDERSTANDING COMPASSION

**EXPLORE**

In the following chapters you will be able to explore the background to compassion, the different views from philosophy, religion and psychology. In addition, you can explore the strengths in more detail as you work through each one.

## Introduction

In this chapter, we will explore what compassion is, what it is not, and how it differs from the similar concepts it is usually associated with. Drawing on philosophy, religion, evolution, spirituality, and psychology it will delve into questions about whether compassion is an emotion, a virtue, a behaviour, or all and more. In this chapter you will learn:

1.  What compassion is
2.  Understanding suffering
3.  What it is not (and how it differs from similar concepts)
4.  Whether it is an emotion, virtue, behaviour, or all three

## What is compassion?

Compassion, what is it? This might seem like an obvious question to answer. However, if we take a deeper look into what compassion means, where it came from and what its roots in society are we will find that it is not so easily

DOI: 10.4324/9781003276425-2

answered and has been discussed and thought about since humans could do so. Compassion has a rich history that stems back as far as early humans came into being. It is important as it can help us thrive, survive, and has benefits for both giver and receiver. It is free to give away and receive from others. We will talk more about the benefits later. But for now, if I was to ask you what compassion was, how would you answer that? Considering that it is such a huge part of healthcare, and an expectation of all practitioners, one would expect to know the answer outright.

Before we look at some definitions of compassion, I'd like you to take some time to think about what compassion means, what it is, what does it entail, and how do we show it? Is it a feeling, behaviour, or more? Write your thoughts below.

_____

_____

_____

_____

_____

Now in the box below, either draw or write what a compassionate practitioner would look like. What would it be about them that would make you say they are compassionate, what characteristics would they show?

---

**BOX 2.1 WHAT A COMPASSIONATE PRACTITIONER LOOKS LIKE**




---

What compassion is, is a question that I have thought about in my career. It became the focus of my Ph.D. research and led to the compassion strengths model within this book. I was quite surprised that even though I felt I had an intuitive understating of compassion, the further I explored this phenomenon the more complex it became. I think it can help us to think about what compassion is, what it looks like, and unpick the differences and similarities between compassion and other similar concepts. Definitions aid in our understanding and can be a useful guide. Let us start at the basics and look at the definitions of compassion.

The literal definition of compassion stems from the two Latin words "Com" (pronounced com-a) and "Pati" (pat-a), which means *"To be with suffering."* This definition has been extended over the years with the Oxford English Dictionary defining compassion as, *"sympathetic pity and concern for the sufferings or misfortunes of others"* The Dalai Lama (1995) suggests that compassion is *"a sensitivity to the suffering of self and others, with a deep commitment to try and relieve it."* Similarly, Gilbert (2009) offers the following definition of compassion as *"a deep awareness of the suffering of another coupled with the wish to relieve it"* Goetz et al. (2010) define it as *"the feeling that arises in witnessing another's suffering that motivates a subsequent desire to help."* Jull (2001) suggests that compassion can be defined as a *"deep response to suffering, and its expression requires action from the compassionate."* Kanov et al. (2004), propose that compassion is dependent on three internal processes: *noticing suffering, an emotional reaction to that suffering, and responding to suffering.* The feelings that are evoked from witnessing suffering can lead to either an unpleasant or pleasant experience of compassion, with the latter most likely to aid in the reduction of another's distress, and the former leading to empathy or compassion fatigue[1]. As you will see further on in this chapter, these processes have been seen and thought about for several years and across many schools of thought. Because of the multifaceted nature of compassion, I define it as

> *The ability to draw on strengths during times of need, utilising them to act in response to suffering or vulnerability, whether that be in the service of self or others.*

What these definitions tell us is that compassion concerns awareness, an emotional response, and any action or set of actions to do something about the suffering. Compassion motivates us to act and strengthens our ability to care. We know from the literature that this is also the same for self-compassion. What there seems little of, is how we achieve awareness, the emotional response that will motivate us forward towards the other, and the behaviours or actions that can alleviate the suffering. But what is suffering anyway, what do we mean by this?

## Suffering

Have you ever stubbed your toe? (Ouch!) Most people have and for a second or two would say that they are suffering. They would instantly be aware of the pain too as I'm sure you have. Sometimes though, what someone is suffering from is not as obvious and the pain one feels is kept hidden under the surface. Equally, you may have been with a friend or patient who is suffering because of their mental health, a form of abuse, the loss of someone close to them, a loss of a job, or rejection. Maybe you or a colleague have felt suffering because of your work. We can all suffer in the workplace with interpersonal relationships, and this can lead to burnout where we all suffer even more.

Suffering can mean anything that causes an individual pain, distress, hardship, or hurtful to them. It is important to remember that each is considered important to that person and should be validated. The point I am making here is that suffering is a relative concept with each experience considered painful to the person. Others may look upon them and think well that is not as bad as they are making out and judge them slightly. We need to think about what others refer to as suffering as exactly that. It is about how they perceive it. This links to being non-judgemental. I find the idea of being non-judgemental quite ridiculous. I say this because we are born to make judgements. This is how we survive in the world. Indeed, it can be the difference between life or death. What I propose instead is wiser judgements. When we catch ourselves making critical judgements about others and indeed ourselves, we must stop and think about why and where that is coming from, and more importantly how can we challenge that judgement using our compassion strengths and change them to a kinder more understanding thoughts and observations. Being overly critical is not good for our well-being, so why do it.

From the loss of a loved one, work related stress, to mental and physical illness, it is very much a part of what makes us human. Suffering is a massive part of life and as much as we would want to eradicate it, I believe we would be better to embrace it with compassion. While some quite rightly see suffering as a dreadful thing, others, especially in spiritual and religious practices, consider it as a gift from the gods, a problem to overcome and a major source of learning, or a guide to some unaddressed issue we have ignored.

We see suffering today on our TVs and various media outlets. In many ways this can make us feel sad and that the world is a horrible place to be. But looking at it another way, we can take inspiration from ancient Greece, as in today's films and literature, where life's tragedies were portrayed in plays so that society could connect to the characters' suffering as a means of developing empathy and compassion for them. This helps to bring us closer to the harsh realities of life, whilst at the same time asking us to question and consider what we could do to show compassion towards our fellow human beings. This serves to remind us that rather than move away, we must lean into our patients and our own suffering and embrace it with the courageous strengths of compassion.

Conversely, pain and suffering can also lead to flourishing and opportunities for self-development. The stories of Martin Luther King and Nelson Mandela are examples of why suffering can sometimes lead to profound change and transformative learning. Therefore, suffering is an opportunity that can lead to growth, and finding ways to take our clients through this to a state of well-being is the goal of therapeutic care. Where a certain amount of suffering can be necessary for the development and growth in sensitivity towards the suffering and compassion for self and others, it should never replace compassion for learning or indeed for suffering's sake. The ends should always justify the means. Equally, Ryan (2010) argues that too much compassion can become crippling, leading to fatigue and ineffective care, while too little makes people seem less human. This shows that the nature and complexity of suffering and compassionate response rely on the understanding of the intensity of both. Knowing how much compassion to give for the problem one presents with, is paramount to the flourishing that comes from alleviating their suffering. As will be discussed later in other chapters, several psychological processes occur before arriving at this conclusion.

Likewise, just like any good thing, too much compassion for another's suffering can be counterproductive to the growth of the sufferer. This creates a paradox in which we then must gauge the right amount of compassion to give to others and ourselves. This is one of the reasons why I consider compassion to be a strength. If we squeeze someone too hard, we will hurt them, but apply the right amount, suffering eases and they and we thrive. In the table below, think about the things we all suffer from (I have provided some examples), and write what you are currently suffering with now, and the intensity of that suffering.

**TABLE 2.1** Things we all suffer from

| Things we can all suffer from | Things I suffer from | Intensity (low/medium/high) |
| --- | --- | --- |
| Loss (even keys or phone) | | |
| Pain | | |
| Anxiety | | |
| Depression | | |
| Financial pressure | | |
| | | |

## What compassion is not

To increase our understanding of compassion, let us now explore what compassion is not. Quite often concepts like kindness, empathy, sympathy, pity, and care can become intermingled with the nomenclature of compassion. Untangling these distinct terms and separating them from each other, allows us to focus on and understand what compassion is.

## Kindness

Compassion and kindness are often mistaken for one another, usually because they share many similarities. Both are associated with helping others. In the Oxford English Dictionary kindness is defined as "the quality of being friendly, generous and considerate." Kindness too is found as a subconstruct of compassion for others and self-compassion and is referred to as a character strength in positive psychology. Whilst compassion and kindness share similar qualities that can be equated with happiness or a positive outcome, they equally have unique properties that make them distinct from each other. For example, kindness does not usually require an emotional reaction to suffering for it to be displayed, and in certain cases, compassion extends far beyond an act of kindness. A kind gesture such as opening the door for someone is not motivated by suffering.

## Empathy

Empathy is another concept normally associated with but distinct from compassion. The psychotherapist Carl Rogers (1975) viewed empathy as a way of being with the other person to understand them more. For Davis (1983) empathy is a multidimensional construct with four distinct elements: perspective taking, fantasy, empathic concern, and personal distress. In a sense, empathy holds the same cognitive and emotional responses that originate in the psychological process of compassion. Yet, because it can be elicited by fantasy such as when reading a book, empathy can be activated in ways that are unique to compassion, in that one is seldom motivated to help a fictional character with their suffering despite wanting to or relating to their story. Research suggests that empathy evolved to serve the species and protect against possible threats and as well as cognitive is underlined by biological and genetic functions (Decety et al., 2015). Conversely, Bloom (2017) claims that although empathy is certainly beneficial to promoting prosocial behaviours, emotional empathy should be used with caution as it can lead to an increase in negative feelings such as burnout and emotion fatigue, poor moral judgement and makes us more prone to biases where we favour one person over the many. Nevertheless, empathy is of particular importance when trying to understand the patient's situation, especially when faced with the crises that bring people into contact with nurses. However, research shows that when there is less emotion involved, practitioners are better able to "feel for" rather than "feel with" their patients suffering and reduce the risk of becoming burned out (Hunt et al., 2017). We will explore burnout in a later chapter and the importance of understanding the distinct types of empathy in the exercises section of this book.

Nevertheless, empathy is a key factor in motivating individuals to act in response to suffering or the needs of others which leads to a compassionate response. It helps us understand the needs of others and connects us to the people we care for. To distinguish the difference between the two concepts, it can help to think of compassion as "empathy with legs." Whereas one can relate to the suffering or needs of another human being and empathise with them during their struggle, compassion forces us to take those vital steps towards helping alleviate that suffering and addressing the patient's needs.

## Sympathy

Sympathy is a concept, yet distinct from compassion and empathy. In most cases, the dictionary definition of sympathy is inaccurately associated with compassion

(Oxford Dictionary). The concept of sympathy was discussed with ethics and morality by the philosophers Hume (1739) and later Smith (1759) in ways like the concept of empathy. For both, sympathy formed part of moral conscience and was a way of experiencing the feelings of another by imagining oneself in their situation. Distinguishing the two concepts Wispé (1986) claims that empathy is a way of knowing the other person and how suffering affects them, while sympathy involves being aware of and concerned for another's suffering. Unlike the compassionate person who feels a deep connection with the suffering, a sympathetic person acknowledges another's suffering and nothing more (Jull, 2001). Still, according to Gilbert (2005) sympathy is a key indicator of compassion as a response to suffering, in the same sense that Smith describes sympathy as the glue that holds people together in times of need.

## Pity

Pity is defined in the Oxford English dictionary as the sympathy or sorrow felt for the sufferings of another. The beginning of compassion can be seen in this definition in that when we first encounter another's suffering, feelings develop concerning another's plight. However, Jull (2001) argues that pity is a fear-based response to the pitier's raised awareness of their vulnerability. Both pity and sympathy can be considered passive, and to a lesser extent empathy too, while compassion is an active endeavour. For example, an individual can show pity by believing they have contributed to alleviating another's suffering without becoming involved in it (Von Dietze & Orb, 2000). According to Brandon (1990), through the combination of arrogance and sympathy centered in smugness and complacency, pity impedes true genuine giving, seeing people as lesser beings. This, according to Von Dietze and Orb (2000), can evoke thoughts of "rather them than me" in practitioners.

Pity and sympathy give rise to our awareness of another's suffering, while empathy helps us understand it. Compassion does all these things but takes it further through action.

## Is compassion an emotion, a virtue, a behaviour, or all three and more?

There is debate in the literature as to whether compassion is an emotional response to suffering, a virtue, a behaviour, or all three. Compassion has been defined as an emotion (Goetz et al., 2010), while others describe it as a multidimensional motivational system (Gilbert, 2009). To answer this question, we shall now explore the various views from philosophy, theology, and psychology. But first, write down your thoughts on this and the reasons for your answer below.

_____

_____

_____

From early philosophical thinkers to religious scholars, evolutionists, and modern-day psychologists, compassion has been a hot topic of debate for years. The earliest reports of compassion can be found in the writings of the ancient philosophers, so we shall start there.

## Philosophical perspectives

Philosophy has always been interested in virtues. Scientific research stems from philosophical points of view, the questions we ask and ponder become hypothesised, evaluated, and either confirmed or rejected. We hear of the virtues being living a life of kindness, goodness, and doing what is right. Aristotle (355–322) gave the first ever conceptual account of compassion (eleos) when speaking of pity as the pain felt by one when seeing the evil put upon another who was not deserving of that misfortune and was someone with whom those witnessing the pain could relate to in some way. From this point on I shall refer to pity as compassion. According to Aristotle's theory, compassion was dependent on three beliefs. First, the suffering is serious. Second, the suffering was not brought on by the person's own doing. Third, those bearing witness to the suffering recognise that they too might also be susceptible to the same kind of anguish (Aristotle, 355–322). Similarly, philosophers argued that compassion should be reserved for a fellow reputable citizen who had fallen from tough times and might respond with thanks upon being pitied (Blowers, 2010). From this idea, we can summarise that compassion includes both feelings and judgements about another's suffering. Hume's (1739, 2003) interpretation was that compassion for another arose out of sympathy for their plight. Hobbes (1968) held a similar position of thought to Aristotle when he said that grief grew from imagining that the adversity of another might also happen to oneself. However, rather than call it pity, He referred to this experience as "compassion," or in the presence of another's suffering, "fellow-feeling."

Later philosophers saw compassion as consisting of the direct participation in the easing of another's suffering regardless of any ulterior motives. For Schopenhauer (2012) compassion was the sole source of all moral actions. Plato, Nietzsche, and Kant believed that "showing" pity towards another was more rational than "feeling" pity for them as in doing so they removed the misery of feeling another's pain (Parkin, 2006). In a similar debate, it is often argued that pity and compassion are based on an emotional rather than a virtuous response to suffering (Carr, 1999).

Likewise, Kant (1774) saw sharing in another's pain as only serving to double the suffering between people. Plato and Nietzsche both proposed that the feelings of compassion and pity use valuable energy that might otherwise be spent helping the individuals heal their wounds (Weber, 2005). For this, Plato (1894) criticised the emotional aspect of compassion other the need to act on our suffering when he said,

*We should take counsel about what has happened, and when the dice have been thrown order our affairs in the way which reason deems best; not, like children who have had a fall, keeping hold of the part stick and wasting time in setting up a howl, but always accustoming the soul forthwith to apply the remedy, rising that which is sickly and fallen, banishing the cry of sorrow by the healing art.* (Plato, 1894, p. 262)

Plato felt that dwelling on misfortunes only served to perpetuate suffering, often referring to it as "irrational," "idle" and "a friend of cowardice" (Plato, 1894).

Nussbaum (1996) argues that the Stoic philosophers were also less in favour of compassion, preferring to see it as an emotion that prevented rational thought. Yet, in Marcus Aurelius' book "Meditations" and other stoic works, there are references throughout to the benefits of helping, and how one should treat their brethren, their community, and others in their community with kindness (Aurelius, 1559). Despite compassion not being discussed as such, the thoughts put forward by the Stoics suggest that compassion or elements of it were a valued virtue that should be developed daily to build the strength of character.

## Religious perspectives

When it comes to compassion, all religious faiths follow the Golden Rule that was first set out by Confucius when he said, "to treat others as you would like them to treat you" (Armstrong, 2011). There are an estimated 5.8 billion people, 84% of the world's population, who have affiliation to religious faith. Christianity, Hinduism, Judaism, Buddhism, and Islam are the largest religious groups in the world today. Religion is often associated with compassion and prosocial behaviours. For example, although Christian texts are inspired by Greek philosophy the process outlined earlier by Aristotle where one might or might not be believed deserving of compassion does not tend to feature.

The bible refers to compassionate acts that require the "right" balance of compassion and intelligence to make a helpful person, as a certain level of intellect is needed to understand another's situation and be moved to action because during this cognitive process a solution to the suffering is found. This is like Buddhism, where one needs only to develop two qualities equally to reach perfection: Compassion [karuna] which stands for qualities of the heart and emotion, such as charity, love, tolerance, kindness, and wisdom [panna] which is the intellectual qualities of the mind. If one or the other is out of balance then the individual either becomes "a good-hearted fool," or a "hard hearted intellect without feelings for others."

Christians often show their compassion through acts of charity, seeing themselves as the conduit between God and his children (Barad, 2007; Feldmeier, 2016). Indeed, studies show that Christians who attended worship show more commitment to their faith, are after humbler and more compassionate, and are more likely to supply emotional support to their friends and family.

The idea of compassion as service to others can be found in other religions. For instance, in Hinduism, God's love, mercy, and compassion stretched far beyond the faith of the believer, even to those who denied God's very existence, while suffering occurs from attachment, and the law of Karma (Whitman, 2007). To connect with God, Hindus believe in debt to nature, to their parents, to friends, to the animals that supply nourishment, the oxygen, and water, and their blessings, and that they must show compassion towards the suffering in humanity through acts of kindness (Sivananda, 1999). The Buddhist tradition also shares the idea that suffering comes from the pointless endeavour of attachment to things outside of self (Harvey, 2000, 2013). Only when this suffering is brought into awareness can one free themselves and become truly engaged in the virtue of compassion for others (Dalai Lama, 1995, 2001). Buddhism is therefore the practice of the Buddha's teachings (Dharmas) that when put into practice all living beings can be liberated from suffering (Gyatso, 2011). In all Buddhist traditions, the spirit of the Buddha embodies compassion and acts of loving-kindness. Loving kindness to rescue all people by whatever means possible, and compassion to suffer with the suffering and be with their illness (Kyokai, 1966).

People of Jewish faith see compassion as a virtue that all are deserving of and that when shown to others can be rewarding. Like the Buddhist idea of wisdom and compassion, engaging in compassionate acts as well as the pursuit of knowledge is encouraged. Compassion is also considered a way of advocating for another in their time of need (Sinclair, 2003). Human vulnerability is met with compassion because of the belief that none could withstand God's wrath alone.

In the Islamic faith, compassion is an essential virtue for all Muslims and is at the centre of their beliefs. Like other scriptures, the Quran speaks of justice and compassion for the poor and unfortunate. For Muslims compassion represents the same virtues as all other religious beliefs and the desire to do something to alleviate suffering in the world, and extend this compassion to all beings (Alharbi & Al Hadid, 2019;Engineer 2001). Judgements such as ego, the colour of skin, ethnicity, interest, and beliefs can all affect how compassion is shown to others but are viewed as being reserved for only Allah, who is the only one who can witness all beings and therefore pass judgement, and so Muslims are encouraged to widen their compassion to all and as far as possible (Engineer 2001).

We can see here that compassion is present throughout and underpins the major world religions and involves more action than feelings. Compassion lies at the heart of each of these traditions as a guiding example of service to others through action more than feeling. Understanding how different ethnic groups understand compassion and suffering is important for both the patient and the practitioner, as each will have a unique perspective that ultimately affects how they give and receive compassionate care.

## Psychological and evolutionary perspectives

Psychology and evolutionary theory have provided us with great insights into how compassion develops and what it is, how is influenced by others, identity, beliefs, and motivations. Research into primate behaviour shows that compassion served as an evolutionary function predating philosophy and religion (DeWall, 1996). In the Descent of Man, Darwin (1879) spoke of kindness and sympathy as being beneficial for reproduction. Most known for suggesting that the survival of the fittest guided evolution, he also wrote that kindness was more important for survival, as it related to flourishing and then more reproduction. More recent views propose that the behaviour of kindness was rewarded with more mating opportunities because altruism was viewed as a positive attribute when raising families (Keltner, 2010). Indeed, social psychologists see compassion as resulting in prosocial behaviours. In an extensive review of the literature, Goetz et al. (2010), concluded that compassion is a unique emotion that evolved specifically to alleviate suffering, help the raising of offspring, mate selection, and cooperative behaviours between groups. Like Aristotle, they suggest that a person goes through a series of psychological processes before deciding of someone is deserving of compassion. Adding further support for this, Stellar et al. (2015) found the vagus nerve, a part of the autonomic nervous system that had evolved to react with compassion when presented with the suffering of another. Indeed, Keltner (2010) suggests that both humans and animals have what he called a "compassionate instinct." So, as well as helping us care for one another it has the added benefit of helping us with our romantic relationships.

The work of developmental psychologist John Bowlby (1969) has shown how attachment and compassionate behaviours can equally have a positive impact on vulnerable children (Mikulincer et al., 2005). Using soothing techniques with a distressed child, helps them form secure attachments and bonds with a caregiver and then has a positive impact on their wellbeing later in life. If you have children or have experience with them, you know that soothing either through words or behaviours such as a hug helps calm them down and feel better when they are upset in most cases. Equally, studies show that even at the age of 18 months, children display compassionate behaviours towards others (Warneken & Tomasello, 2006). In support of this, Gilbert (2015) proposes that compassion is very much a part of the human capacity that evolved through caring motivational systems and social characteristics, cultivated through cognitive, societal, social identity and cultural processes that brought benefits to both the tribe and the mind of the individual. He names three emotional regulation systems (soothing, seeking, and threat) that we use to regulate our emotions and needs. Our threat system keeps us safe from harm, and our drive system guides us to seek out that which we need to survive. Problems can occur when either or both systems go into overdrive. For example, too much threat leads to anxiety and worry, while increased drive can lead to addictive behaviours. To counter these issues, the soothing system needs to be activated. This is achieved through self-compassion, or compassion from others. It also tells us that compassion has an emotional element as well as the consequent behaviours that follow to alleviate distress.

Alternative theories suggest that gene selfishness can translate into individualism for the sole benefit of the gene rather than the organism. In this way, a limited amount of altruism is present but only to serve the selfish goal of the gene (Dawkins, 1976). People may also react compassionately to the suffering of others to seem moral and just in the eyes of others and gain reciprocal favours (Brosnan & De Waal, 2002). As Goffman (1959) proposed, humans present themselves to the rest of society as an actor would on stage, to project an image that is desirable for work-related reasons or to form relationships and gain information about others. However, Grinde (2005) argues that through their actions human beings can adjust their way of thinking to see how compassion helps them as well as society. For some, compassion is a virtue that leads the individual to what they believe to be a just and moral life; one that brings them happiness and a sense of meaning. For example, someone who follows a certain religious doctrine might be motivated by the need to serve God, whilst psychologically, showing compassion and helping others makes people feel good about themselves (Cornelius, 2013).

What do you think now? Is it a behaviour, an emotion, a virtue or all three? How do these ideas affect your thinking about compassion? What motivates your compassion? Write your thoughts below.

_____

_____

_____

_____

_____

As it is often seen today, there are mixed views about compassion being either an emotion, behaviour, virtue or all the above. It stands as a reminder that compassion is not always understood as straightforward, both for its emotional aspect and expressed behaviours. However, we can take from this then that compassion includes all, as it includes emotions, rationality, cognition, and action. It involves a mixture of awareness, empathy, and behaviours that help alleviate the suffering of others. These things form the building blocks of the compassion strengths model that guides the practices in this book which we will look at in more detail later. Healthcare practitioners rely not only on their competence and technical skills but the emotional abilities such as empathy when they deliver compassionate care (Kerasidou et al., 2021).

Knowing what compassion is and is not can help us understand and show when it is being demonstrated in practice. It can help us move away from a judgement-based reaction to diverse ways of being compassionate. The point here is that compassion can be shown in many ways, and to recognise this is to become more aware of what compassion is and how it is actioned in practice.

## Conclusion

In exploring and unpacking what it is, from the definitions we can see that compassion involves three distinct parts of awareness, motivation, and action. First, through awareness and understanding of our own and others' suffering, through a mindful judgement based on wisdom and empathy for the severity of suffering, we are motivated toward a compassionate response. The final aspect is the act or acts of compassion that are shown to alleviate the suffering or pain felt by another. We have learned that this relies on similar concepts such as kindness, sympathy, and empathy. From the different views across philosophy, religion, and psychology you have learned that compassion is both a virtue, emotion, and behaviour. The question then becomes what do these characteristics look like, and how can you develop and bring them into your practice. We will explore these questions and how compassion works in healthcare systems in greater depth in the next chapter.

What these behaviours and emotions are, form the core of this book. The compassion strengths that you will learn about have each of the emotions and behaviours to create a compassionate outcome. In the next chapter, we will explore what hinders and enables compassion to flourish in healthcare systems. In later chapters, we will answer questions about whether we are born with compassion or if it is a learned trait. And if so, how to do practitioners learn to be compassionate or develop their innate compassion in ways that help them and the people they work with in healthcare. I believe very strongly that compassion is just as if not more important for healthcare as it is for all of humankind, but even if we are born with compassion, it still needs to be nurtured for the patient and client.

What have you learned that you did not know before?

_____

_____

_____

_____

_____

## Note

1 The term compassion fatigue has been heavily contested by researchers in the field of neuropsychology with many arguing that it is empathy distress fatigue and not compassion that people suffer from. We will explore this in more depth in the next chapter.

## References

Alharbi, J., & Al Hadid, L. (2019). Towards an understanding of compassion from an Islamic perspective. _Journal of clinical nursing_, 28, 1354–1358.

Armstrong, K. (2011). Twelve Steps to a Compassionate Life. Bodley-Head.

Aurelius, M. (1559, 2006). _Meditations_. London: Penguin.

Barad, J. A. (2007). The understanding and experience of compassion: Aquinas and the Dalai Lama. *Buddhist-Christian Studies, 27*(1), 11–29.

Bloom, P. (2017). *Against empathy: The case for rational compassion.* London: Random House.

Blowers, P. M. (2010). Pity, empathy, and the tragic spectacle of human suffering: Exploring the emotional culture of compassion in late ancient Christianity. *Journal of Early Christian Studies, 18*(1), 1–27.

Bowlby, J. (1969, 1984). *Attachment and loss: (Vol. 1) Attachment.* Harmondsworth: Penguin.

Brandon, D. (1990). Zen in the Art Of Helping. Routledge.

Brosnan, S. F., & De Waal, F. B. (2002). A proximate perspective on reciprocal altruism. *Human Nature, 13*(1), 129–152.

Carr, B. (1999). Pity and compassion as social virtues. *Philosophy, 74*(3), 411–429.

Cornelius, E. (2013). The motivation and limits of compassion. *HTS Theological Studies, 69*(1), 1–7.

Dalai Lama (2001). *The compassionate life.* London: Simon and Schuster.

Dalai Lama (1995). *The power of compassion.* London: Thorsons.

Darwin, C. (1879, 2004). *The descent of man.* London: Penguin.

Davis, M. H. (1983). Measuring individual differences in empathy: Evidence for a multi-dimensional approach. *Journal of Personality and Social Psychology, 44*(1), 113–126. 10.1037/0022-3514.44.1.113

Dawkins, R. (1976). *The selfish gene.* Oxford: Oxford University press.

Decety, J. (2015). The neural pathways, development and functions of empathy. *Current Opinion in Behavioral Sciences, 3,* 1–6.

De Waal, F. B. M. (1996) *Good natured: The origins of right and wrong in humans and other animals.* Harvard: Harvard University Press.

Engineer, A. A. (2001). On the concept of compassion in Islam. *Global Religious Vision, 2,* 1–11.

Feldmeier, R. (2016). "As Your Heavenly Father is Perfect": The God of the Bible and Commandments in the Gospel. *Interpretation, 70*(4), 431–444.

Gilbert, P. (2005). *Compassion: Conceptualisations, research and use in psychotherapy.* London: Routledge.

Gilbert, P. (2009). *The compassionate mind: A new approach to life's challenges.* London: New Harbinger Publications.

Gilbert, P. (2015). The evolution and social dynamics of compassion. *Social and Personality Psychology Compass, 9*(6), 239–254.

Goetz, J. L., Keltner, D., & Simon-Thomas, E. (2010). Compassion: An evolutionary analysis and empirical review. *Psychological Bulletin, 136*(3), 351–374. 10.1037/a0018807

Goffman, E. (1959). *The presentation of self in everyday life.* London: Penguin.

Grinde, B. (2005). Darwinian happiness: Can the evolutionary perspective on well-being help us improve society? *World Futures, 61*(4), 317–329.

Gyatso, K. (2011). *Modern Buddhism: The path of compassion and wisdom.* Glen Spey, NY: Tharpa Publications US.

Harvey, P. (2000). *An introduction to Buddhist ethics: Foundations, values and issues.* London: Cambridge University Press.

Harvey, P. (2013). *The selfless mind: Personality, consciousness and nirvana in early Buddhism.* London: Routledge.

Hobbes, T. (1968). *Leviathan.* Harmondsworth: Penguin.

Hume, D. (1739, 2003). *A treatise of human nature.* Mineola, NY: Dover Publications.

Hunt, P. A., Denieffe, S., & Gooney, M. (2017). Burnout and its relationship to empathy in nursing: A review of the literature. *Journal of Research in Nursing, 22*(1–2), 7–22.

Jull, A., (2001). Compassion: A concept exploration. *Nursing Praxis in New Zealand*, *17*, 16–23.

Kanov, J. M., Maitlis, S., Worline, M. C., Dutton, J. E., Frost, P. J., & Lilius, J. M. (2004). Compassion in organizational life. *American Behavioral Scientist*, *47*(6), 808–827.

Kant, I. (1774). *The metaphysics of morals*. Cambridge: Cambridge University Press.

Keltner, D. (2010). The Compassion Instinct. In D. Keltner, J. Marsh, & J. A. Smith (Eds), *The compassionate instinct: The science of human goodness* (pp. 8–15.). London: Norton & Company.

Kerasidou, A., Bærøe, K., Berger, Z., & Brown, A. E. C. (2021). The need for empathetic healthcare systems. *Journal of Medical Ethics*, *47*(12), e27–e27.

Kyokai, B. D. (1966). *The teaching of Buddha*. Tokyo: Kosaido.

Mikulincer, M., Shaver, P. R., Gillath, O., & Nitzberg, R. A. (2005). Attachment, caregiving, and altruism: Boosting attachment security increases compassion and helping. *Journal of Personality and Social Psychology*, *89*(5), 817–839.

Nussbaum, M. (1996). Compassion: The basic social emotion. *Social Philosophy and Policy*, *13*(1), 27–58.

Parkin, A. (2006). You do him no service': An exploration of Pagan almsgiving. In *Margaret Atkins and Robin Osborne. Poverty in the Roman World* (pp. 61–63). Cambridge: Cambridge University Press.

Plato (1894). *The republic*. Translated by B. Mineola Jowett. Dover.

Rogers, C. R. (1975). Empathic: An unappreciated way of being. *The Counselling Psychologist*, *5*(2), 2–10. 10.1177%2F001100007500500202

Ryan, T. (2010). Aquinas on compassion: Has he something to offer today? *Irish Theological Quarterly*, *75*(2), 157–174.

Schopenhauer, A. (2012). The World as Will and Representation, Vol. 2. Dover Publications Inc.

Sinclair, D. B. (2003). Advocacy and compassion in the Jewish tradition. *Fordham Urban Law Journal*, *31*, 99.

Sivananda, S. (1999). All About Hinduism (Shivanandanagar, India: Divine Life Society), 1947. Online version (www.dlshq.org/download/hinduismbk.Htm). Accessed April 2016.

Smith, A. (1759, 2009). *Theory of moral sentiments*. London: Penguin.

Stellar, J. E., Cohen, A., Oveis, C., & Keltner, D. (2015). Affective and physiological responses to the suffering of others: Compassion and vagal activity. *Journal of Personality and Social Psychology*, *108*(4), 572–582.

Von Dietze, E., & Orb, A., (2000). Compassionate care: A moral dimension of nursing. *Nursing Inquiry*, *73*, 166–174. 10.1046/j.1440-1800.2000.00065.x

Warneken, F., & Tomasello, M. (2006). Altruistic helping in human infants and young chimpanzees. *Science*, *311*(5765), 1301–1303.

Weber, M. (2005). Compassion and pity: An evaluation of Nussbaum's analysis and defence. *Ethical Theory and Moral Practice*, *7*(5), 487–511.

Whitman, S. M. (2007). Pain and suffering as viewed by the Hindu religion. *The Journal of Pain*, *8*(8), 607–613.

Wispé, L. (1986). The distinction between sympathy and empathy: To call forth a concept, a word is needed. *Journal of Personality and Social Psychology*, *50*(2), 314–321.

# 3

# COMPASSION IN HEALTHCARE ORGANISATIONS

## Introduction

Building on the earlier chapter we will explore compassion in healthcare systems. This chapter will outline the benefits of compassion to patients, staff, and healthcare organisations. It will explore the different factors that both hinder and enable compassion to flourish, and the outcomes for both student and staff professional quality of life, such as burnout and compassion fatigue, and what can be done to move beyond the suffering of self, others and the wider healthcare systems practitioners work in to improve wellbeing for all. This chapter will cover:

1. The benefits of compassion in healthcare organisations
2. What hinders and enables compassion to flourish in healthcare
3. The outcome of both for students and staff professional quality of life
4. How to move beyond patients, staff, and organisational suffering and improve wellbeing.

## The benefits of compassion to healthcare organisations

There is no other place like a healthcare organisation where people work together to alleviate the suffering of others. Doctors, nurses, psychologists, social workers, midwives, allied health, leaders, volunteers, and administrators the world over, all working towards the same goal of offering compassionate care to those in need. Understandably, students and practitioners feel compelled and pulled toward working in healthcare because they want to show compassion and help others. In fact, one only needs to search, and you will find compassion at the very heart of healthcare policy and procedure all over the world.

DOI: 10.4324/9781003276425-3

Compassion as many benefits. Studies in positive psychology suggest that practicing compassion and engaging in compassionate acts helps increase happiness, and self-esteem, and reduce the symptoms of depression, along with other positive benefits (Mongrain et al., 2011). For example, compassion has the power to transform the person and move them beyond their suffering (Lomas, 2015), and can heal both the giver and the receiver (Stone, 2008). This is important, as we will see later when we talk about compassion fatigue. Compassion has also been shown to aid social relationships. When individuals show compassion and kindness to others, they form similar emotional bonds to those found in friendships (Crocker & Canevello, 2012). In healthcare systems, compassion has benefits for patients/service users, clients, and staff including relationships with self and others, and the organisation where healthcare students and practitioners' work. We will now look at each one of these areas in more detail. Before we do that write down what you think are the key benefits of compassion to your patients/clients/service users, you (your staff/colleagues), and the organisation you work in.

To patients

_____
_____
_____
_____
_____

To staff

_____
_____
_____
_____
_____

To your organisation

_____
_____
_____
_____
_____

## Patients

Compassion helps the patient in many ways. It can help reduce patient anxiety in those seeking medical attention as well as improve patient satisfaction and the relationship between patient and practitioner, and better health outcomes which are all linked to a higher standard of care (Pehlivan & Güner, 2020). Compassion fosters a human connection between patient and practitioner and the recognition of our common humanity. When treated with compassion, patients feel listened to and understood. It can help improve patients' mental health and physical health, leading to calmness and increased wellbeing. Interventions for helping patients develop compassion such as Compassion Focused Therapy, Mindful Self-Compassion, and Compassion Cultivation Training have been created with promising results for an entire range of mood disorders, and traumas, and are particularly beneficial for those high in self-criticism (Kirby, 2017).

## Staff (self-other)

For staff, compassion for both self and others is associated with increased well-being, greater job and compassion satisfaction, and job retention, plus lower burnout. A compassionate rather than intimidating approach to patients makes them more responsive and helps stimulate openness to provide detailed information to nurses and physicians that could help with their care (Sinclair et al. 2016a). Compassion between colleagues also improves working relations between staff members, students, and the care team. Supporting each other and working together for the benefit of the patient and client care, helps foster collective compassion for self and other relations. This in turn helps the organisation people work in.

## Organisations

Work-related stress can cost healthcare organisations billions in lost time and even more for staff illness. Despite the finical issues, more importantly, when stress-related issues are not addressed this can lead to mental health issues among staff. Avoidance of duties and loss of care become organisational symptoms of the stress caused by working in such places, and ultimately patients suffer more. Therefore, not only does compassion help the organisations in creating harmony and satisfaction among staff, but it also has financial benefits by helping reduce absenteeism and stress-related illness among staff. Rewarding compassion in staff is also associated with increased compassion for patients (Lown et al., 2019). Organisations should foster a collective compassion, where you collaborate with colleagues and managers within your place of work, find your strengths and when combined, you can all work together to create a compassionate workplace for each other and your patients and their families. Compassion should flow down and up and all around.

## What hinders and enables compassion to flourish in healthcare

While it is an expectation that all students and practitioners should be compassionate, this is not always the case. As we have become to know, compassion is more complex than it seems on the surface. Various factors can both hinder and enable compassion in equally complex healthcare systems. These can differ among different professions, experiences, and specialisations but generally they can be internal, such as motivation, self-care practices, personality, age, and gender, or external like working conditions, support from others, feeling supported by your organisation, having a positive role model, the clinical environment and the people you care for, or support (Jones et al., 2016). As compassion is a social mentality, how one perceives compassion depending on their culture influences how it is showed (Cheon et al., 2013). For instance, coming from an individualistic culture where self-expression, individualism independence, and the pursuit of personal goals, are less likely to be motivated to show compassion to others compared to a collective culture that supports togetherness, harmony, and interdependence within groups. However, studies show with people from a collective culture have less compassion for others, and more self-compassion (Steindl et al., 2020). We can categories the enablers and hinderers of compassion into four domains that relate to the personal, workplace, interpersonal (relational), and educational factors. Let's begin with the workplace. But before that reflect on these questions below.

What might hinder or enable your compassion, now, in the past, and the future?

_____

_____

_____

_____

_____

## Workplace factors

We spend a larger number of hours of our life in the workplace. The workplace is often considered the primary barrier and facilitator of compassion (Singh et al., 2018). They are places where we get to bear witness to the experiences of others and practice our compassion. Under the right conditions, the workplace is conducive to compassion, whilst at other times they can drain the very life out of our resources and limit our desire for a compassionate response. The work healthcare workers do is psychically, emotionally, and cognitively demanding which can drain wellbeing and increase burnout. Various stressors can result in the normally kind practitioner detaching emotionally from patients restricting their motivation to be compassionate to themselves and others. Newly qualified students experience various impediments to delivering compassion, such as the negative attitude of the staff who had adopted a clinical approach to care, whereas supportive environments enable compassion to flourish (Cole-King & Gilbert, 2011; Horsburgh et al., 2013).

Compassion is at the forefront of any healthcare profession as the essential quality needed to deliver effective care. Working in understaffed fast paced environments, which are target driven, with a heavy workload, at risk from harm either from contagious illnesses, violent or harmful patients, with little autonomy in our work with little or no support from others has an impact on compassion. Indeed, the perceived threat of the organisation can prevent healthcare workers from showing compassion (Henshall et al., 2018). A common response to not showing compassion is not having the time to because of these fast-paced workplaces. I argue that this shows a lack of understanding of compassion and how it can be achieved through the small things just as easily as the big. Compassion can be seen in the small moments through a smile, a gentle understanding touch, or as simple as making someone a cup of tea (Durkin, 2022). Furthermore, now because of Covid-19, not only is the work more challenging but the masks worn by staff and students have become another thing that limits the ability to show compassion and empathy. They make it increasingly difficult to express compassion and communicate to others the understanding and desire to help.

Yet, in contrast, in workplaces where staff are supported, have strong collegial networks, have manageable workloads, are led by helpful leaders, and are part of a supportive team, compassion can flourish (Dewar & Nolan, 2013). Nurses who feel supported, valued, and have their concerns substantiated both in and outside of the workplace, are better equipped to deliver compassionate care. Practitioners that feel respected and understood tend to show compassion more than those who do not. Which makes sense. We are more likely to act with compassion or in a positive way when we feel heard and feel valued. Equally, and for students having a role model to learn about compassion helps, while people in certain roles and more experienced professionals tend to have more compassion. For example, psychiatrists tend to have more compassion than general practitioners, and experienced doctors report fewer barriers to compassion than their younger inexperienced counterparts (Fernando & Consedine, 2017). Indeed, Figley (1995) suggests that younger caregivers are more susceptible to compassion fatigue and burnout than their more experienced counterparts. Whereas nurses generally experience fewer barriers to compassion but greater workplace-related barriers than physicians (Dev et al., 2018).

Social psychology and social science in general, have long argued that environments rather than an individual's decision to choose, explains why people do what they do. The fundamental attribution error is one prime example that is used to suggest that behaviour is falsely assumed to be a result of an individual's personality and not the circumstances practitioners find themselves in. This was shown in Zimbardo's Stanford Prison Experiment where seemingly "good" participants were assessed on personality and behaviour traits before participation in the study, but still showed cruelty towards others. The study showed that it was situational variables that influenced behaviour and not the attitudes or beliefs of the participants. However, recent studies into this have shown that the participants in Zimbardo's infamous study were coerced into doing the dreadful things, showing that when a senior figure pressures someone to do something they are more likely to do it even if it goes against their better nature (Haslam et al., 2019). Without the pressure from an authority, people are more likely to act in ways that are more aligned with kindness and compassionate. Likewise, Tierney et al. (2018), propose that healthcare organisations should take responsibility for allowing compassion to flourish, rather than lay the blame solely at the feet of staff. There are allegations that healthcare students and staff work in complex bureaucratic organisations where external factors that suppress individual moral values are to blame for failures of care in practice. However, inadvertently, this line of argument makes a compelling case for the need to nurture the strengths of compassion in those that work under such conditions, and papers like this should not be used to disregard personal factors such as character, personality, disposition, or human agency. Using the environment to explain the reasons why people are not able to show compassion, excludes them from taking responsibility for their actions because it is the situation and not them that caused this. Social psychology would argue that it is interventions that need to change to take away the barriers to being compassionate. Yet this puts intervention over the intention and a person's will to show compassion no matter what and under the harshest of circumstances. Thus, intention trumps intervention all the time, because people have free will and with strength can make the choice to be compassionate over anything else.

## Personal factors

Within the working environment is another environment - a human being who has been shaped and influenced by their experiences, the world around them, and the people in it. Personal factors such as beliefs (self-fulfilling prophecy), values, personal attributes, exposure to suffering, coping strategies, level of compassion and empathy, resilience to stress, distress tolerance, control over self and situation, self-care and compassion strategies, feeling competent, age, gender, personality, socio-economic status, experience, and motivation all combine to hinder or enable our compassion. Issues at home that affect our focus and wellbeing, can also change, and hinder the compassion we show. While these are common and valid reasons, there are also ways to overcome them. For example, if one is not confident with their skills, they can learn and develop the strengths needed to show compassion. Or, if it is stress or burnout that is taking its toll on the practitioner's emotions and ability to do their work with compassion, then taking responsibility to look after the self with self-care activities that help alleviate these emotional barriers can help too. Of course, people do become victims of their environment, but they are also the captains of their future and can take themselves out of their current situation.

Compassionate behaviour is also influenced by the individual values and characteristics of the healthcare student or professional (Nijboer & Van der Cingel, 2018). Personality traits can both hinder and enable compassion. In one study of intensive care unit nurses, extraversion was associated with compassion satisfaction, neuroticism, and agreeableness linked to burnout and compassion fatigue (Barr, 2018). Whereas paediatric nurses who scored high on extraversion, agreeableness, conscientiousness, and were more engaged in outdoor activities had greater compassion satisfaction, those with less emotional stability and who were single were more at risk of compassion fatigue (Chen et al., 2018). Egotistical caregiving where the practitioner cares more about their role and ability in the caring process, rather than care itself can also prevent compassion (Singh et al., 2018). Personal attributes such as a humbler approach, and being approachable, kind, and honest can help support compassion.

Other psychological factors such as beliefs and attitudes towards particular people can have a profound effect on the subsequent behaviour. The Francis Report (2013) claimed that the occurrences at Mid-Staffordshire NHS Trust were because of staff following orders. Acting on one's beliefs to challenge a current immoral and malevolent authority can be helped by an autonomous state or hindered by an agentic state, in which a person does not take responsibility for their actions and acts as an agent for another's a will, which is usually someone in a position of power. Conversely, an autonomous state refers to when people direct and take full responsibility for their behaviour (Milgram, 1974). Therefore, a practitioner who is showing a lack of compassion may do so because they are under strict orders to only perform their clinical duty, and nothing more. Acquiescing to authority in this way could make the nurse unable to present a fully human response when tending to another human being, thus ostensibly showing them to be lacking in compassion. This type of conformity could also be understood as a coping strategy that novice practitioners adopt to cope with conflicting personal goals to keep their compassion values and organisational goals. However, it is those in Milgram's study and indeed practice in general, who do not follow blindly the commands of a senior figure when faced with another suffering as a result. This was found to be true for nurses, where some challenged rather than conformed to the dissonance between their values and conflicting realities in practice, and by doing so increased the motivation to sustain their compassionate behaviours (Nijboer & Van der Cingel, 2018). This is not to dismiss the fact that both individual and environmental factors play a mutual role in human behaviour. Instead, it serves as a reminder that the harshest of environments will test even the most compassionate practitioner and unsupportive leadership, and that no amount of training will change those who do not possess the intrinsic qualities of compassion.

A person's beliefs can be greatly influenced by the psychological benefits that completing a certain behaviour might have on an individual. This is illustrated in a future thinking mindset that looks forward toward goals rather than back to mistakes. Compassion leads the individual to what they believe to be a just and moral life; one that brings them happiness and a sense of meaning (Jull, 2001). For example, someone who follows a certain religious doctrine might be motivated by the need to serve God, whilst psychologically, showing compassion and helping others makes people feel good about themselves (Cornelius, 2013).

Compassion can also become self-fulfilling. It can go both ways too. False and positive beliefs about ability, skills, deserving for compassion, and giving to others can deeply change someone's beliefs about their capabilities. Led to believe they are capable; students are more likely to achieve remarkable things based on the expectations of their peers. While those that do not have the same positive beliefs imposed on them will be more likely to not perform to their full abilities.

(Rosenthal & Jacobson, 1968). An example of this is when based on a "one-time" incident a student is labelled as being lazy by their manager. Others respond to this label and the student starts to accept the label and begins to show 'lazy behaviours. Similarly, students and practitioners can be affected by a self-fulfilling prophecy, which leads them to believe that they are not compassionate nor can become compassionate in their work. A potential consequence of this type of self-belief is that they lose their motivation to learn or develop their compassion. These feelings of incompetence can take away valuable cognitive load that could be spent on showing compassion. With the reports of poor care and negative media coverage of these incidents, practitioners and students must remain strong and keep their compassion strengths.

## Interpersonal (relational)

Interpersonal factors refers to the people we work with, whether that is the patient, their families, or colleagues and managers, and how we relate to and interact with them, and them with us, through communication, and the aim of a common language of compassion. Developing positive relationships with patients, their families, and colleagues can help to facilitate compassion. Patients who are polite, less aggressive, respectful, and take initiative enable compassion, while those that are considered difficult, rude, aggressive, and resistant to care, hinder compassion (Fernando & Consedine, 2014). These factors can lead to either like or contempt for patients, which again can help or hinder the compassion shown to them. As was mentioned in the last chapter, we run through a series of psychological assessments of the other in which we consider them as being deserving or undeserving of our compassion. We might conceive the homeless intravenous drug user as being less deserving of our compassion than the cancer patient. Sometimes it can be hard to show compassion in these situations just like it is difficult to keep our compassion with aggressive or threatening patients and families. Our critical judgements can cloud our ability to show compassion to them. This is where our wisdom can shine, and we should go forward with a wiser judgement to deepen our understanding of the reasons why they behave that way. Communication, and finding a common language, empathy, and openness to connecting with patients can help ease this understanding and support their emotional, personal, and psychological needs. However, we can also experience gratitude and thanks from patients and their families. This leads to feelings of compassion satisfaction, which then further enables compassion for others. Knowing that what you did was effective becomes a reward cycle of compassion which begets compassion satisfaction which begets more compassion, that benefits all involved in the care process.

## Educational/training

While compassion is at the forefront of healthcare organisations, there seems to be little in the way of teaching and learning about compassion. Barriers to this include a proposed lack of understanding of what compassion means for practitioners in healthcare settings, as well as the promotion of practice training. Most educational programs are provided in healthcare settings with very few offered at the student level, even though it is recommended that healthcare students need more training for compassion. These also tend to focus on practical skills more than compassion (Bray et al., 2014). Nurses in particular report that the transition to practice does not support the integration of compassion learned in education (Sinclair et al., 2016c). Research also tells us that medical students and less experienced healthcare practitioners experience greater barriers to compassion due to a lack of training resources (Dev et al., 2018). Training courses that have been evaluated seem to focus more on preventing compassion fatigue and burnout while improving resilience through mindfulness practices. When training attends to the qualities and attributes of a compassion practitioner it has the power to equip practitioners with the skills that enable compassion to flourish and empower patients and staff alike. Gilbert (2010) propose that Compassionate Mind Training could be introduced into the curriculum for healthcare students and staff to reduce self-critical judgements and support the regulation of emotions that alleviate their suffering, and their patients. Studies show that this approach can indeed help practitioners become more compassionate towards themselves and others (Beaumont et al., 2021, McVicar et al., 2021), and protect them from the negative consequences of working in stressful environments.

## Individual and collective responsibility

Overall, it is both an individual and collective responsibility to remove the barriers to compassion and enable students and practitioners to offer compassionate care to others and themselves (Lown, 2015). This helps remove blame from practitioners while encouraging them to take responsibility for learning about and to show compassion. Nevertheless, have we have seen, all individuals including students and staff have agency for who they choose to be aware of, empathise with, and address someone else's suffering. While organisations share the responsibility, compassion for personal and individual transformation is needed for staff to overcome the self-imposed restrictions that disenable them and their application of compassion.

## Outcomes of both students and staff

What are the positive outcomes of (Self/Other) compassion for you?

_____

_____

_____

_____

_____

What are the negative outcomes of compassion for you?

_____

_____

_____

_____

_____

**TABLE 3.1** The positive and negative outcomes of compassion

| Positive | Negative |
| --- | --- |
| Compassion Satisfaction | Empathy/Compassion Fatigue |
| Wellbeing | Burnout |
| Self-compassion | Secondary Traumatic Stress |

The joint outcomes of these complex factors can usually be grouped into positive and negative experiences. At one end of the spectrum, you have compassion fatigue, secondary traumatic stress, and burnout. And on the other, compassion satisfaction, and well-being. All are equally affected by personal and organisational factors and can affect the compassion shown to self and others.

The most common outcomes of work, personal, relational, and educational aspects of healthcare systems that impede or enable practitioners' compassion are stress-related such as burnout, secondary traumatic stress, and compassion fatigue, and positive such as compassion satisfaction and wellbeing. Compassion fatigue and burnout have become synonymous with caring for others, and quite often we hear more about these concepts and experiences than we do about compassion itself. In a recent review of the literature Ondrejková, N., & Halamová (2022), found that high rates of compassion fatigue, secondary traumatic stress, and burnout were prevalent across helping professions and were highest in doctors. We will explore how both are an outcome of work, personal and educational systems, as well as how they too can feedback into these same systems and become hinders and enablers of compassion in practice.

## Compassion fatigue/secondary traumatic stress

Joinson (1992) coined the term "compassion fatigue" after noticing that a growing number of nurses report feelings of exhaustion after work with patients. Adding to this, Figley (1995) referred to compassion fatigue as the "cost of caring" that resulted from experiencing another's suffering. Compassion fatigue can occur when seeing the suffering of others and showing compassion towards them leads to feelings of fatigue if we are not able to help them. The term has been used as a less stigmatising way to describe secondary traumatic stress (STS). This has been likened to the experience of post-traumatic stress but happens vicariously after listening to and being with another's story of trauma. Figley defines STS as "*the stress deriving from helping others who are suffering or who have been traumatised.*" Secondary traumatic stress is probably more common as a response to being with another's trauma. Studies exploring healthcare workers' experiences across the globe during the Covid-19 pandemic found that over 40% suffered from STS (Orrù et al., 2021). This is more prevalent in healthcare students and practitioners who are exposed to direct trauma, and especially those who work with emergencies. Nurses and paramedics are more exposed to indirect trauma which leaves them more prone to developing STS (Ogińska-Bulik et al., 2021).

However, compassion fatigue has come under scrutiny lately for not properly addressing the true nature of what it means to be compassionate, and the positive outcomes associated with helping others.

## Compassion or empathic distress fatigue?

There have been recent developments in neuropsychology that now challenge the idea of compassion fatigue instead of proposing that it is empathy that creates fatigue and the feelings and symptoms that are usually associated with compassion fatigue. What this research and others argue is that compassion is rewarding and is driven by a desire to help others and thus motivates good feelings. Equally, because compassion includes the self, having and more to the point using our self-compassion helps alleviate any distress we might experience from working with difficult stories, and enables us to continue being compassionate. As you will see in the next chapter, in developing the compassion strengths scale, I found that compassion strengths predict lower reported burnout. Self-care and the understanding of the different types of empathy can help regulate the emotional distress that occurs when being present with another's experience.

As was mentioned earlier in this chapter compassion is a powerful antidote to suffering for both the giver and receiver. This brings into question how compassion fatigue can exist when compassion is invigorating. McClelland & Vogus (2021) found, engaging in compassionate acts created vitality rather than fatigue among healthcare practitioners. The same can be said for empathy in that there are different kinds of empathy we can employ with patients. For example, cognitive empathy is less likely to lead to empathy fatigue or burnout, while emotional empathy will (Bloom, 2017). Similarly, if we practice self-compassion, or take part in self-care strategies that improve our mood and well-being then we can project ourselves from compassion fatigue or variations of it.

## Burnout

Burnout is a state of emotional and physical exhaustion that occurs from working in stressful roles for a prolonged period. It has been referred to as workplace depression due to the similarities between symptoms and the effects it has on people. Students and practitioners experience this more when working in a stressful and unsupportive environment. It is mainly comprised of three factors: emotional exhaustion, depersonalisation, and personal accomplishment (Maslach & Jackson, 1984). Burnout is perpetuated by poor working conditions, heavy workloads, and negative workplace cultures (Christiansen et al., 2015; De Zulueta, 2013). As a result of working in these conditions, nursing students in particular experience negative self-judgements which in turn compromise their compassion for others (Durkin et al., 2016), making them more susceptible to depression (Cornwell & Goodrich, 2009). In the US, healthcare workers are twice as at risk of suffering from burnout as the general population (Shanafelt et al., 2012). Compassion fatigue and burnout exist across a diverse range of practitioner groups, including professionals and students (Beaumont et al., 2016a & b; Cavanagh et al., 2020; Durkin et al., 2016), but are seen more in nurses due to their heavy workloads and working conditions.

Although it might seem like it is only you who is going through this experience, it might help you to know that you are not alone. It is estimated that around 20% of the working population suffers from burnout (Lindblom et al., 2006). Around one-tenth of the global nursing, the population is said to have experienced an elevated level of burnout (Woo et al., 2020). An international study involving 33, 659 nurses found that almost half (42%) reported feeling burned out (Aiken 2002). There has been an increased number of practitioners reporting burnout and emotional exhaustion during the Covid-19 pandemic (Chen et al., 2021), with over 50% of 184 healthcare workers reporting emotional exhaustion and depersonalisation (Orrù et al., 2021).

## Compassion satisfaction

Compassion satisfaction is the positive feeling practitioners experience from their work helping others, which leads to improved engagement, pleasure, and fulfilment (Stamm, 2009). Adapting to stressful situations in this way has been likened to a form of resilience (Russell & Brickell, 2015). Nurses who treat and alleviate the suffering of others, experience compassion satisfaction (Burridge et al., 2017). It is associated with an increase in compassion for others among nursing students (Durkin et al., 2016). Therefore, compassion becomes satisfying for the practitioner, which then increases the compassion they show to patients, which then leads to more satisfaction, and thus a positive loop of compassion and compassion satisfaction appears in the student and healthcare worker.

## Wellbeing

Wellbeing is defined as being in a state of contentment, and happiness, having a good outlook on life with little distress, and good mental and physical health. It is important for reasons relating to positivity in the individual, across teams, and for productivity in the workplace. People with higher well-being often report added benefits of improved relationships, more cooperation, living longer, better physical, and mental health, stress less, and being more prosocial (Huppert & So, 2013). Suffering and well-being are part of being human, and both deserve equal attention. Self-care can help students and practitioners achieve their optimal level of wellbeing and compassion strength.

## Self-compassion/kindness

Self-compassion and positive psychology interventions are effective means of alleviating the symptoms of work-related stress, and improving wellbeing, flourishing, happiness, and optimism. Self-compassion is an evidenced based approach to being kinder to yourself. It is associated with less critical judgement, reduced burnout, and increased well-being and compassion satisfaction among students and healthcare practitioners. We know from research that as a self-care practice, self-compassion can potentially thwart burnout and compassion fatigue (Beaumont et al., 2016a, b; Durkin et al., 2016). There are certain personal costs involved in the devotion of compassion to others, yet the ability to cope with stressful situations is positively related to compassion and negatively to feelings of distress. Distress tolerance is a key feature of compassion for self and others, in that one learns to adjust their ability to manage distress through mindful thought, self-soothing, and action so that they can address the other more fully (Gilbert, 2010). Self-compassion and developing a compassionate mind are both forms of self-care that can help towards this endeavour.

Having looked at the varied factors in more detail we can see what both hinders and enables compassion to flourish in healthcare systems. For instance, the professional quality of life of students and practitioners can affect their ability to show compassion. Stress-related issues such as burnout, secondary traumatic stress, and stress buffers such as compassion satisfaction, self-compassion, and wellbeing either enable or hinder compassion.

Learning how to recognise barriers to compassionate care coupled with the self-care strategies that protect students' and practitioners from compassion fatigue and burnout enables individuals to navigate through their working environments and become more compassionate practitioners. For instance, self-care helps foster a greater feeling of compassion satisfaction, which can also help nurses who are battling compassion fatigue and burnout (Hinderer et al., 2014) and has been shown to reduce compassion fatigue and improve satisfaction among social workers (Cuartero & Campos-Vidal, 2019). More on this later.

## Conclusion

Compassion in healthcare can be hindered or it can be enabled through a wide range of a range of factors. This shows how complex the systems both work and personal are and how they interact with our compassion. While the working environment can affect our ability to show compassion, it does not and cannot hinder it completely. This is based on an outdated behaviourist theory that reward and punishment decide one's actions. The truth of the matter is that we are cognitive beings that can make choices that decide our fate and future directions. Just like those in the classic study in obedience by Stanley Milgram, not all chose to follow orders and deliver the shocks, or let their situation affect the compassion they have for others. So, while we may suffer from burnout because of the workplace, or compassion fatigue/secondary trauma and stress because of the nature of our work, we can do something about that and improve our mood and situation through the development of our compassion strengths, both at the individual and organisational level. These factors should be viewed as barriers to overcome rather than complete and impenetrable barriers. Hence the reason each aspect of the compassion model you will learn about are called strengths. Yet, under the right conditions, and with guidance for self-care and practice that help their beliefs and values, students and professionals can learn how to flourish as compassionate practitioners. In the next chapters, we will explore the compassion strengths model.

What have you learned that you did not know before?

_____

_____

_____

_____

_____

# References

Aiken, L. H., Clarke, S. P., Sloane, D. M., Sochalski, J., & Silber, J. H. (2002). Hospital nurse staffing and patient mortality, nurse burnout, and job dissatisfaction. *JAMA*, *288*(16), 1987–1993.

Barr, P. (2018). The five-factor model of personality, work stress and professional quality of life in neonatal intensive care unit nurses. *Journal of Advanced Nursing*, *74*(6), 1349–1358. 10.1111/jan.13543

Beaumont, E., Bell, T., McAndrew, S., & Fairhurst, H. (2021). The impact of compassionate mind training on qualified health professionals undertaking a compassion-focused therapy module. *Counselling and Psychotherapy Research*, *21*(4), 910–922.

Beaumont, E., Durkin, M., Hollins Martin, C. J., & Carson, J. (2016a). Measuring relationships between self-compassion, compassion fatigue, burnout and well-being in student counsellors and student cognitive behavioural psychotherapists: a quantitative survey. *Counselling and Psychotherapy Research*, *16*(1), 15–23. 10.1002/capr.12054

Beaumont, E., Durkin, M., Martin, C. J. H., & Carson, J. (2016b). Compassion for others, self-compassion, quality of life and mental well-being measures and their association with compassion fatigue and burnout in student midwives: A quantitative survey. *Midwifery*, *34*, 239–244. 10.1016/j.midw.2015.11.002

Bloom, P. (2017). *Against empathy: The case for rational compassion*. London: Random House.

Bray, L., O'Brian, M.R., Kirton, J., Zuairu, K., & Christiansen. (2014). The role of professional education in developing compassionate practitioners: A mixed methods study exploring the perceptions of health professionals and pre-registration students. *Nurse Education Today, 34*(3), 480–486.

Burridge, L. H., Winch, S., Kay, M., & Henderson, A. (2017). Building compassion literacy: Enabling care in primary health care nursing. *Collegian, 24*(1), 85–91. 10.1016/j.colegn.2015.09.004

Cavanagh, N., Cockett, G., Heinrich, C., Doig, L., Fiest, K., Guichon, J. R., ... & Doig, C. J. (2020). Compassion fatigue in healthcare providers: A systematic review and meta-analysis. *Nursing Ethics, 27*(3), 639–665.

Chen, C., & Meier, S. T. (2021). Burnout and depression in nurses: A systematic review and meta-analysis. *International Journal of Nursing Studies, 124*, 104099.

Chen, Y. P., Tsai, J. M., Lu, M. H., Lin, L. M., Lu, C. H., & Wang, K. W. K. (2018). The influence of personality traits and socio-demographic characteristics on paediatric nurses' compassion satisfaction and fatigue. *Journal of Advanced Nursing, 74*(5), 1180–1188. 10.1111/jan.13516

Cheon, B. K., Mrazek, A. J., Pornpattananangkul, N., Blizinsky, K. D., & Chiao, J. Y. (2013). Constraints, catalysts and coevolution in cultural neuroscience: Reply to commentaries. *Psychological Inquiry, 24*(1), 71–79.

Christiansen, A., O'Brien, M. R., Kirton, J. A., Zubairu, K., & Bray, L. (2015). Delivering compassionate care: the enablers and barriers. *British Journal of Nursing, 24*(16), 833–837. 10.12968/bjon.2015.24.16.833

Cole-King, A., & Gilbert, P. (2011). Compassionate care: The theory and the reality. *Journal of Holistic Healthcare, 8*(3), 29–37.

Cornelius, E. (2013). The motivation and limits of compassion. *HTS Theological Studies, 69*(1), 1–7.

Cornwell, J., & Goodrich, J. (2009). Ensuing compassionate care in hospital. *Nursing Times. 105*(15), 14–16.

Crocker, J., & Canevello, A. (2012). Consequences of self-image and compassionate goals. *Advances in Experimental Social Psychology, 45*, 229–277.

Cuartero, M. E., & Campos-Vidal, J. F. (2019). Self-care behaviours and their relationship with satisfaction and compassion fatigue levels among social workers. *Social Work in Health Care, 58*(3), 274–290.

Dev, V., Fernando III, A. T., Lim, A. G., & Consedine, N. S. (2018). Does self-compassion mitigate the relationship between burnout and barriers to compassion? A cross-sectional quantitative study of 799 nurses. *International Journal of Nursing studies, 81*, 81–88. 10.1016/j.ijnurstu.2018.02.003

Dewar, B., & Nolan, M. (2013). Caring about caring: Developing a model to implement compassionate relationship centred care in an older people care setting. *International Journal of Nursing Studies, 50*, 1247–1258. 10.1016/j.ijnurstu.2013.01.008

De Zulueta, P. (2013). Compassion in healthcare. *Clinical Ethics, 8*(4), 87–90.

Durkin, M., Beaumont, E., Martin, C. J. H., & Carson, J. (2016). A pilot study exploring the relationship between self-compassion, self-judgement, self-kindness, compassion, professional quality of life and wellbeing among UK community nurses. *Nurse Education Today, 46*, 109–114.

Durkin, M., Gurbutt, R., & Carson, J. (2022). Effectiveness of an online short compassion strengths course on nursing students compassion: A mixed methods non-randomised pilot study. *Nurse Education Today, 111*, 105315.

Fernando III, A. T., & Consedine, N. S. (2017). Barriers to medical compassion as a function of experience and specialization: Psychiatry, pediatrics, internal medicine, surgery, and general practice. *Journal of Pain and Symptom Management, 53*(6), 979–987.

Fernando III, A. T., & Consedine, N. S. (2014). Beyond compassion fatigue: The transactional model of physician compassion. *Journal of Pain and Symptom Management, 48*(2), 289–298.

Figley, C. R. (1995). Compassion fatigue: Toward a new understanding of the costs of caring. In B. H. Stamm (Ed.), *Secondary traumatic stress: Self-care issues for clinicians, researchers, and educators* (pp. 3–28). Baltimore, MD: The Sidran Press.

Francis, R. (2013). *Report of the Mid Staffordshire NHS Foundation Trust: Public Inquiry.* London: The Stationery Office (TSO).

Gilbert, P. (2010). An introduction to compassion focused therapy in cognitive behavior therapy. *International Journal of Cognitive Therapy, 3*(2), 97–112.

Haslam, S. A., Reicher, S. D., & Van Bavel, J. J. (2019). Rethinking the nature of cruelty: The role of identity leadership in the Stanford Prison Experiment. *American Psychologist, 74*(7), 809.

Henshall, L. E., Alexander, T., Molyneux, P., Gardiner, E., & McLellan, A. (2018). The relationship between perceived organisational threat and compassion for others: Implications for the NHS. *Clinical Psychology & Psychotherapy, 25*(2), 231–249.

Hinderer, K. A., VonRueden, K. T., Friedmann, E., McQuillan, K. A., Gilmore, R., Kramer, B., & Murray, M. (2014). Burnout, compassion fatigue, compassion satisfaction, and secondary traumatic stress in trauma nurses. *Journal of Trauma Nursing, 21*(4), 160–169.

Horsburgh, D., & Ross, J. (2013). Care and compassion: the experiences of newly qualified staff nurses. *Journal of Clinical Nursing, 22*(7–8), 1124–1132. 10.1111/jocn.12141

Huppert, F. A., & So, T. T. (2013). Flourishing across Europe: Application of a new conceptual framework for defining well-being. *Social Indicators Research, 110*(3), 837–861. 10.1007/s11205-011-9966-7

Joinson, C. (1992). Coping with compassion fatigue. *Nursing, 22*(4), 116–118.

Jones, J., Winch, S., Strube, P., Mitchell, M., & Henderson, A. (2016). Delivering compassionate care in intensive care units: nurses' perceptions of enablers and barriers. *Journal of Advanced Nursing, 72*(12), 3137–3146. 10.1111/jan.13064

Jull, A. (2001). Compassion: A concept exploration. *Nursing Praxis in New Zealand, 17,* 16–23.

Kirby, J. N. (2017). Compassion interventions: The programmes, the evidence, and implications for research and practice. *Psychology and Psychotherapy: Theory, Research and Practice, 90*(3), 432–455.

Lindblom, K. M., Linton, S. J., Fedeli, C., & Bryngelsson, I. L. (2006). Burnout in the working population: Relations to psychosocial work factors. *International journal of behavioral medicine, 13*(1), 51–59.

Lomas, T. (2015). Self-transcendence through shared suffering: An intersubjective theory of compassion. *Journal of Transpersonal Psychology, 47*(2).

Lown, B. A. (2015). Compassion Is a Necessity and an Individual and Collective Responsibility Comment on "Why and How Is Compassion Necessary to Provide Good Quality Healthcare?". *International journal of health policy and management, 4*(9), 613–614. 10.15171/ijhpm.2015.110

Lown, B. A., Shin, A., & Jones, R. N. (2019). Can organizational leaders sustain compassionate, patient-centered care and mitigate burnout?. *Journal of Healthcare Management, 64*(6), 398–412.

Maslach, C., & Jackson, S. E. (1984). Burnout in organizational settings. *Applied Social Psychology Annual*, *5*, 133–153.

McClelland, L. E., & Vogus, T. J. (2021). Infusing, sustaining, and replenishing compassion in health care organizations through compassion practices. *Health Care Management Review*, *46*(1), 55–65.

McVicar, A., Pettit, A., Knight-Davidson, P., & Shaw-Flach, A. (2021). Promotion of professional quality of life through reducing fears of compassion and compassion fatigue: Application of the Compassionate Mind Model to Specialist Community Public Health Nurses (Health Visiting) training. *Journal of Clinical Nursing*, *30*(1–2), 101–112.

Milgram, S. (1974). *Obedience to authority: An experimental view*. New York: Harper & Row.

Mongrain, M., Chin, J. M., & Shapira, L. B. (2011). Practicing compassion increases happiness and self-esteem. *Journal of Happiness Studies*, *12*(6), 963–981. 10.1007/s10902-010-9239-1

Nijboer, A. A., & Van der Cingel, M. C. J. M. (2018). Compassion: Use it or lose it? A study into the perceptions of novice nurses on compassion: A qualitative approach. *Nurse Education Today*, *72*, 84–89.

Ogińska-Bulik, N., & Michalska, P. (2021). Psychological resilience and secondary traumatic stress in nurses working with terminally ill patients—The mediating role of job burnout. *Psychological Services*, *18*(3), 398.

Ondrejková, Natália, & Halamová, Júlia (2022). Prevalence of compassion fatigue among helping professions and relationship to compassion for others, self-compassion and self-criticism. Health & Social Care in the Community, 30, 1680–1694. 10.1111/hsc.13741

Orrù, G., Marzetti, F., Conversano, C., Vagheggini, G., Miccoli, M., Ciacchini, R., ... & Gemignani, A. (2021). Secondary traumatic stress and burnout in healthcare workers during COVID-19 outbreak. *International Journal of Environmental Research and Public Health*, *18*(1), 337.

Pehlivan, T., & Güner, P. (2020). Compassionate care: Benefits, barriers and recommendations. *Journal of Psychiatric Nursing*, *11*(2), 148–153.

Rosenthal, R., & Jacobson, L. (1968). Pygmalion in the classroom. *The Urban Review*, *3*(1), 16–20.

Russell, M., & Brickell, M. (2015). The "Double-Edge Sword" of human empathy: A unifying neurobehavioral theory of compassion stress injury. *Social Sciences*, *4*(4), 1087–1117.

Shanafelt, T. D., Boone, S., Tan, L., Dyrbye, L. N., Sotile, W., Satele, D., ... & Oreskovich, M. R. (2012). Burnout and satisfaction with work-life balance among US physicians relative to the general US population. *Archives of Internal Medicine*, *172*(18), 1377–1385.

Sinclair, S., Norris, J. M., McConnell, S. J., Chochinov, H. M., Hack, T. F., Hagen, N. A., McClement, S., & Bouchal, S. R. (2016a). Compassion: a scoping review of the healthcare literature. BMC Palliative Care, 15, 6–6.

Sinclair, S., McClement, S., Raffin-Bouchal, S., Hack, T. F., Hagen, N. A., McConnell, S., & Chochinov, H. M. (2016b). Compassion in health care: An empirical model. *Journal of Pain and Symptom Management*, *51*(2), 193–203. 10.1016/j.jpainsymman.2015.10.009

Sinclair, S., Torres, M.-B., Raffin-Bouchal, S., Hack, T. F., McClement, S., Hagen, N. A., & Chochinov, H. M. (2016c). Compassion training in healthcare: what are patients' perspectives on training healthcare providers? BMC. Medical Education, 16, 169–169.

Singh, P., Raffin-Bouchal, S., McClement, S., Hack, T. F., Stajduhar, K., Hagen, N. A., ... & Sinclair, S. (2018). Healthcare providers' perspectives on perceived barriers and facilitators of compassion: Results from a grounded theory study. *Journal of Clinical Nursing, 27*(9–10), 2083–2097.

Stamm, B. H. (2009). Professional quality of life: Compassion satisfaction and fatigue version 5 (ProQOL). [2011-03-20]. http://www.isu.edu/bhstamm

Steindl, S. R., Yiu, R. X. Q., Baumann, T., & Matos, M. (2020). Comparing compassion across cultures: Similarities and differences among Australians and Singaporeans. *Australian Psychologist, 55*(3), 208–219.

Stone, D. (2008). Wounded healing: Exploring the circle of compassion in the helping relationship. *Humanistic Psychologist, 36*(1), 45–51.

Tierney, S., Bivins, R., & Seers, K. (2018). Compassion in nursing: Solution or stereotype? *Nursing Inquiry, 26*, e12271.

Woo, T., Ho, R., Tang, A., & Tam, W. (2020). Global prevalence of burnout symptoms among nurses: A systematic review and meta-analysis. *Journal of Psychiatric Research, 123*, 9–20.

# 4

# COMPASSION STRENGTHS

## Introduction

In this chapter, you will be introduced to the Compassion Strengths model. As well as exploring questions about whether compassion can be taught it will provide an overview of the guidelines for developing each of the eight strengths and their significance to healthcare students and practitioners. In this chapter you will gain insight into:

1. If compassion can be taught in healthcare
2. Motivation and mindset
3. The five Ws to consider when learning about compassion
4. The Compassion Strengths Model

## Can compassion be taught, or can you learn to be compassionate?

Before we go any further, I would like you to take a moment to reflect on this important question about compassion in healthcare. What do you think – can it be taught, or can you learn how to show it in practice? Write your answers and reasons why below.

_____

_____

_____

_____

_____

DOI: 10.4324/9781003276425-4

This is a question that has raised an eyebrow and debate when asked. In the literature and among professionals, it is almost seen as a given that those working in healthcare are automatically and naturally compassionate. However, if this was the case why do we have issues around a lack of compassion or poor patient care? You might rightly be thinking, stress, burnout, and all the other things previously mentioned that impact compassion. But as has also been discussed, a more integrated approach to compassion that includes self as well as others, and that compassion itself can be energising. If this is the case, then what else could be causing this? We would also be able to say with certainty what compassion was and how it was demonstrated in practice with patients, self, and others. Yet, when asked many people find it hard to pin down and often confuse compassion with empathy and kindness. A few passionately believe that it cannot be taught. This seems myopic to presume that one could not learn about or be taught ways in which they could develop their natural or even gain a better understanding of compassion and implement it into the work they do. I believe that while it is more unlikely that you can teach compassion, you can help people learn how to develop and apply it to their work. Like clinical skills, which we might consider hard skills, students and practitioners can learn about what we might call soft skills of compassion. But do not be fooled. Compassion is by no means a soft skill, nor is it soft. As I have said, compassion requires strength on the practitioner's part to develop, maintain and demonstrate to self and others. The problem, I think is that the behaviours of compassion have not properly been understood or evidenced in healthcare to the point they can be taught to students and practitioners.

Indeed, in healthcare staff, there is evidence that compassion can be taught, both on an individual level with self-compassion, and for the other through many different programmes. Students and practitioners with an innate ability for compassion can learn to deepen their skills and strengths to be compassionate. Studies show that compassion meditation training can increase awareness and engagement with suffering (Weng et al., 2018), and increase positive emotions in relation to distress (Klimecki et al., 2013). Comparable results have been found with healthcare workers who reported increased job satisfaction and self-compassion after taking part in an eight-week course for cultivating compassion (Scarlet et al., 2017). Healthcare practitioners agree and report that innate compassion behaviours can be taught and developed and that they should be implemented into training (Sinclair et al., 2020). In my research, where I developed a short online course to teach compassion strengths, we found that nursing students experienced greater improvement in, communication, connection, interpersonal skills, competence, character, and empathy. Participants in this study talked about deepening their understanding of compassion and seeing each strength as contributing to better patient outcomes and their wellbeing (Durkin et al., 2022).

## Mindset and motivation

In positive psychology, there is a theory about how we approach learning and problems called Mindset. This is based on our beliefs in our abilities and wants.

According to this theory, two types of mindsets can determine how we approach learning and intelligence. They are growth and fixed mindsets. Developed by Carol Dweck (2006), mindset proposes that someone who has a fixed mindset believes that they cannot change and will not seek out opportunities for growth as they already believe that the knowledge and skills they have are fixed. People can also become fixed if they believe that they are not capable of learning anything new. On the other hand, individuals with a growth mindset will be more motivated to learn new things and put in more effort because they believe that they can. A fixed mindset is contained in a deterministic view of the world, while a growth mindset is based on free will and the humanistic approach to individuals overseeing their life and learning. Mindset is associated with self-compassion and motivation (Breines et al., 2012). This makes sense as if we try and fail at a task, treating ourselves with compassion counteracts any negative feeling and reminds us that we did our best and can try again.

## What mindset do you have?

Do you think that you can change, learn, and grow, or do you think that your skills and knowledge of compassion are fixed and cannot change?

_____

_____

_____

_____

_____

## Intrinsic and extrinsic motivation

We are motivated by different things. In helping professions this can be purely altruistic or in certain instances, egotistical motivations. Most would want to do good because it is the right thing. Intrinsically we know that it is. While we can argue that it is for the other, it is equally hard to dismiss the fact that one can feel good when helping and therefore helping others helps us gain those good feelings. This is not a terrible thing. Alternatively, others are motivated by pure ego. They want to be seen as good people and be liked by others. Guided by this extrinsic motivation they do things to help themselves more than others. In their seminal paper titled "Shitty Nursing – the new norm", Richards and Borglin (2019), claim that there is a serious problem with nursing care, which indicates a lack of motivation to be compassionate, with some nurses blaming external factors for this. Like earlier examples, they argue that nurses should take more responsibility for their actions and always demonstrate compassion, especially when caring for patients. This argument applies to all healthcare professions. Therefore, it is important to think about the motivation behind wanting to learn about compassion.

How motivated do you feel on a scale of 1 (not much), to 10 (very much) to learn about compassion?

_____

_____

_____

_____

_____

## Motivation to want to develop compassion

Motivation is a key factor in learning about a topic or set of behaviours. Think about some of the things you have wanted to learn, such as learning how to drive. I am sure there were many reasons for you wanting to do this, such as the freedom driving brings, or the joy of owning a car. This would have no doubt motivated you to go through all the challenges and fun elements of learning how to drive. Knowing why can help give us the motivational boost we need to learn a new skill and change our behaviour. Also, consider what might be holding you back and treat that part of yourself with self-kindness and compassion. Self-compassion is a great motivator. To help with this, the five W's can help prompt you towards the reasons why you want to learn about compassion.

## The five Ws for learning about compassion that can help motivate you

This approach was developed with healthcare professionals, students, and educators in several focus groups and interviews. Collectively, everyone agreed that these are the questions to ask yourself when thinking about why you want to learn about compassion. These questions can guide and motivate you towards your goals and help you see how you can develop your compassion strengths. Take time to think about each question and reflect on your answers.

## Why do I want to learn about compassion strengths?

Understanding your reasons for why you want to learn about compassion can be highly motivating. It can be helpful if you are honest with yourself about this. This helps shape your thinking towards the benefits of compassion and why it is important for the work you do. Write your answer to this below.

_____

_____

_____

_____

_____

## What can I (do I want to) learn about compassion?

This question is good if you are thinking about what new skills you can use to develop your compassion. It could be that you focus more on compassion for others and want to learn how you can take care of yourself too. You might want to learn new skills and ways of demonstrating compassion. You might understand compassion but want to learn how to apply this knowledge to practice. You may have years of experience but not the actual formal training in what compassion is. This can either confirm what you already practice or provide you with added information that you can implement into your work.

_____

_____

_____

_____

_____

## How can I learn about compassion strengths?

In thinking about the diverse ways, you can learn about compassion, such as simulation, education, observation, and of course this book and many like it, you can explore several ways of learning about compassion. This book is a helpful guide for the different elements of compassion, and each strength can be explored further with the exercises and links to relevant resources.

_____

_____

_____

_____

_____

## From whom can I learn about compassion strengths?

We can learn about compassion from different people in our personal and professional lives. The people around us can teach us about compassion. Patients, service users, and clients are a primary source of learning about what works with compassion. Equally, our family, strangers, loved ones, colleagues, and educators all play a part in our development and can contribute to our knowledge of compassion.

_____

_____

_____

_____

_____

## Where can I learn about compassion strengths?

Work and educational settings are two of the most beneficial and integral places for learning about compassion. In line with learning from others, these environments not only provide the stimulus for knowledge, but the opportunity to discuss debate, and develop our compassion through daily interactions and reflective practices. What we learn in theory can be applied to practice with the two contributing to the collective understanding of compassion in a healthcare setting.

_____

_____

_____

_____

_____

## Why compassion is a strength

Why strengths? This is a good question that can be answered with several reasons why the aspects of compassion you will be introduced to are considered strengths. Like the definition, to be with suffering, compassion takes strength to endure suffering whether that is someone else's or your own, and the strength to do something about it. This is sometimes referred to as distress tolerance (Gilbert, 2009). The first reason is that during the research that was used to develop the model, participants referred to being compassionate as requiring strength due to the sometimes-difficult nature of the work. The second refers to how each can be cultivated with consistent work and exercise but can also be affected by the work or other things going on in the person's life. It is wrong to assume that practitioners do not have compassion, as though it is something that one either does or does not have and cannot be developed. Compassion takes practice and commitment to the continuous growth of each strength.

Like the muscles of the body that can be worked on, but equally can become fatigued over time, or prone to injury due to overuse or lack of experience, so too compassion. When one feels an imbalance, the whole does not function as it should. Therefore, for students and practitioners to become proficient in their daily exercise of compassion, like an exercise in a gym, guidance and a regular training schedule can help them build on the strengths they already have and make stronger those that need more attention.

## The compassion strengths model

In Chapter 2 we looked at different definitions of compassion. In healthcare compassion shares similar definitions in that are about being aware of and wanting to alleviate patient suffering and improve their wellbeing. Similarities with this definition can be found in most healthcare professions around the world (Gilbert, 2009; Perez-Bret et al., 2016; Seppala et al., 2014; Sinclair et al.,

2016a; Zaragozá et al., 2021). Compassion can be expressed in healthcare as the emotions and behaviours that allow for the understanding of suffering such as empathy, connection, and communication, coupled with the actions of competency-based practices that alleviate it and increase well-being in patients (Sinclair et al., 2018). The international charter for Human Values in Healthcare has compassion as one of its fundamental values that can be demonstrated through the capacities of care, empathy, respect, curiosity genuineness, self-reflection, motivation to help, flexibility in relationships, acceptance, and altruism (Rider et al., 2014).

The earlier chapter looked at how healthcare practitioners maintain their compassion. Showing empathy, connecting to and seeing the humanity in patients, while observing their distress tolerance, and developing self-care strategies to foster resilience act as enablers for compassion to flourish (Baguley et al., 2020). This adds to the argument for a holistic model of compassion that considers these factors as contributing to compassionate behaviour for self as well as others. Wilkes and Wallis (1998) propose that compassion can be actualised through communication, competence, providing comfort, commitment, having concern for patients, consciousness, confidence, and courage. In support of this, Walker et al. (2016) suggest that compassion becomes easier to teach when it is broken down into manageable segments. We can see that there is a common language of compassionate behaviours, emotions, and cognitive expressions that span everywhere across the healthcare professions. Although compassion is a core element of healthcare, its underlying behaviours have not yet been fully realised. This is where the compassion strengths model comes in. By breaking compassion down into its parts, we can learn about what compassion entails and become more compassionate by putting the knowledge of each into practice and combining them. It is well known that focusing on something gives us more of what we attend to, so by becoming aware of each compassion strength we are more likely to develop them.

As described in the definition of compassion, action is what separates compassion from other similar concepts such as empathy and sympathy. This of course helps practitioners understand just what it is they must do or the behaviours they can engage in to show compassion. To aid with this the compassion strengths model consists of, empathy, communication, self-care connection, interpersonal skills, clinical competence, and engagement.

## The eight compassion strengths across healthcare professions

The Compassion Strengths Model was developed through a systematic review of the literature, interviews, focus groups, and statistical modelling with patients, students, practitioners, and educators. It draws on other research in healthcare and combines elements of compassion that may seem obvious to the reader but are unique in that this model brings them all together. It is considered more holistic because it includes competency and self-care. While this model was

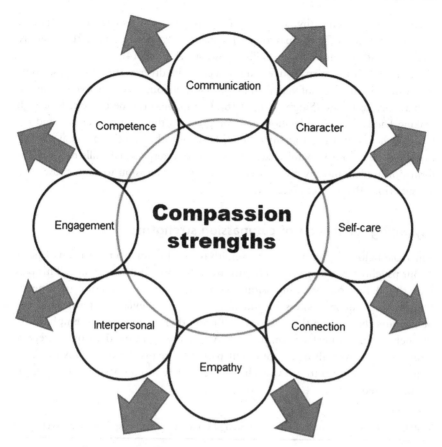

**FIGURE 4.1**   The compassion strengths model

originally developed with nurses, the factors and behaviours that contribute to the compassion strengths can be generalised to other student and practitioner groups as they can be found in many healthcare professions. Similarities are also found in research with healthcare and nursing staff and students (Papadopoulos & Ali, 2016).

For example, nurses, midwives, physicians, operating theatre workers, radiologists, and psychologists all demonstrate one or more of the compassion strengths in this book. Engagement, character, and connection have been identified as attributes of compassion in healthcare (Taylor et al., 2017). As was found with radiation therapists, who considered the behaviour of compassion to consist of connection, character, and communication (Taylor & Hodgson, 2020). Likewise intensive and palliative care staff named connection, character and going above and beyond with small acts of kindness (Roze des Ordons et al., 2019). Midwives report that compassion is expressed through meaningful connections, character, empathy, communication, interpersonal skills, and supportive care during childbirth (Krausé et al., 2020). In acute mental health, practitioners refer to kindness, empathy, warmth, caring, respect, and patient centred among the characteristics of a compassionate mentality (Crawford et al., 2013) that are enhanced with communication skills (Crawford et al., 2014).

From the patient perspective, and especially in diverse ethnic groups, communication in the form of verbal and non-verbal actions such as active listening is seen as compassionate (Singh et al., 2018). Compassion can be expressed through shaking hands, but consideration must be given to the person's cultural and religious beliefs as in Islam touching the other sex is forbidden (Babaei et al., 2016). Equally, a kind and hopeful character as well as interpersonal skills to share information understandably are viewed as showing compassion towards those who are suffering (Brooten et al., 2013).

## Psychological aspects of compassion strengths

The table below shows how each strength relates broadly to the various aspects of our psychology, such as our cognitions, emotions, and behaviours. This taps into the definition of compassion, with cognitions and emotional aspects, encouraging our awareness of and motivation to alleviate suffering and the behaviours that enable this. As you will note, there is more of an emphasis on the behavioural aspect of compassion. A few are in more than one category while others cover all of the different parts of our psychology. This can give you more insight into how each of the different compassion strengths is demonstrated.

**TABLE 4.1** Classification of compassion strengths in each different aspect of our psychology

| Compassion Strength | Behaviour | Emotion | Cognitive |
| --- | --- | --- | --- |
| Empathy | | – | – |
| Self-care | – | – | – |
| Character | – | – | – |
| Communication | – | – | – |
| Competence | – | | – |
| Engagement | – | | |
| Interpersonal | – | | – |
| Connection | – | – | – |

## Conclusion

In this chapter, we have explored the compassion strengths that you can develop. The 5 Ws were outlined to help stimulate your thinking around what and how you can learn about compassion. You have been introduced to the Bolton Compassion Strengths Indicator and been given the chance to measure your compassion. In the next chapter, we will go through a series of reflective and practical exercises that can help you develop each of your strengths.

What have you learned that you did not know before?

_____

_____

_____

_____

_____

## References

Babaei, S., Taleghani, F., & Kayvanara, M. (2016). Compassionate behaviours of clinical nurses in Iran: An ethnographic study. *International Nursing Review, 63*(3), 388–394.

Baguley, S. I., Dev, V., Fernando, A. T., & Consedine, N. S. (2020). How do health professionals maintain compassion over time? Insights from a study of compassion in health. *Frontiers in Psychology, 11,* 564554.

Breines, J. G., & Chen, S. (2012). Self-compassion increases self-improvement motivation. *Personality and Social Psychology Bulletin, 38*(9), 1133–1143.

Brooten, D., Youngblut, J. M., Seagrave, L., Caicedo, C., Hawthorne, D., Hidalgo, I., & Roche, R. (2013). Parent's perceptions of health care providers actions around child ICU death: What helped, what did not. *American Journal of Hospice and Palliative Medicine®, 30*(1), 40–49.

Crawford, P., Brown, B., Kvangarsnes, M., & Gilbert, P. (2014). The design of compassionate care. *Journal of Clinical Nursing, 23,* 3589–3599. 10.1111/jocn.12632

Crawford, P., Gilbert, P., Gilbert, J., Gale, C., & Harvey, K. (2013). The language of compassion in acute mental health care. *Qualitative Health Research, 23*(6), 719–727.

Durkin, M., Gurbutt, R., & Carson, J. (2022). Effectiveness of an online short compassion strengths course on nursing students compassion: A mixed methods non-randomised pilot study. *Nurse Education Today, 111,* 105315.

Dweck, C. S. (2006). *Mindset: The new psychology of success.* Random House Publishing Group.

Gilbert, P. (2009). *The compassionate mind: A new approach to life's challenges.* London: New Harbinger Publications.

Klimecki, O. M., Leiberg, S., Lamm, C., & Singer, T. (2013). Functional neural plasticity and associated changes in positive affect after compassion training. *Cerebral Cortex, 23*(7), 1552–1561.

Krausé, S. S., Minnie, C. S., & Coetzee, S. K. (2020). The characteristics of compassionate care during childbirth according to midwives: A qualitative descriptive inquiry. *BMC Pregnancy and Childbirth, 20*(1), 1–10.

Papadopoulos, I., & Ali, S. (2016). Measuring compassion in nurses and other healthcare professionals: An integrative review. *Nurse Education in Practice, 16,* 133–139.

Perez-Bret, E., Altisent, R., & Rocafort, J. (2016). Definition of compassion in healthcare: A systematic literature review. *International Journal of Palliative Nursing, 22*(12), 599–606.

Richards, D. A., & Borglin, G. (2019). 'Shitty nursing' – The new normal?. *International Journal of Nursing Studies, 91,* 148–152.

Rider, E. A., Kurtz, S., Slade, D., Longmaid III, H. E., Ho, M. J., Pun, J. K. H., ... & Branch Jr, W. T. (2014). The International Charter for Human Values in Healthcare: An interprofessional global collaboration to enhance values and communication in healthcare. *Patient Education and Counselling, 96*(3), 273–280.

Roze des Ordons, A. L., MacIsaac, L., Everson, J., Hui, J., & Ellaway, R. H. (2019). A pattern language of compassion in intensive care and palliative care contexts. *BMC Palliative Care, 18*(1), 1–9.

Salvador Zaragozá, A., Soto-Rubio, A., Lacomba-Trejo, L., Valero-Moreno, S., & Pérez-Marín, M. (2021). Compassion in Spanish-speaking health care: A systematic review. *Current Psychology*, 1–20.

Scarlet, J., Altmeyer, N., Knier, S., & Harpin, R. E. (2017). The effects of Compassion Cultivation Training (CCT) on health-care workers. *Clinical Psychologist, 21*(2), 116–124.

Seppala, E. M., Hutcherson, C. A., Nguyen, D. T., Doty, J. R., & Gross, J. J. (2014). Loving-kindness meditation: A tool to improve healthcare provider compassion, resilience, and patient care. *Journal of Compassionate Health Care, 1*(1), 1–9.

Sinclair, S., Hack, T. F., McClement, S., Raffin-Bouchal, S., Chochinov, H. M., & Hagen, N. A. (2020). Healthcare providers perspectives on compassion training: A grounded theory study. *BMC Medical Education, 20*(1), 1–13.

Sinclair, S., Hack, T. F., Raffin-Bouchal, S., McClement, S., Stajduhar, K., Singh, P., ... & Chochinov, H. M. (2018). What are healthcare providers' understandings and experiences of compassion? The healthcare compassion model: A grounded theory study of healthcare providers in Canada. *BMJ Open, 8*(3), e019701.

Sinclair, S., Norris, J. M., McConnell, S. J., Chochinov, H. M., Hack, T. F., Hagen, N. A., ... & Bouchal, S. R. (2016a). Compassion: A scoping review of the healthcare literature. *BMC Palliative Care, 15*, 193–203. 10.1186/s12904-016-0080-0

Singh, P., King-Shier, K., & Sinclair, S. (2018). The colours and contours of compassion: A systematic review of the perspectives of compassion among ethnically diverse patients and healthcare providers. *PloS One, 13*(5), e0197261. 10.1371/journal.pone.0197261

Taylor, A., & Hodgson, D. (2020). The behavioural display of compassion in radiation therapy: Purpose, meaning and interpretation. *Journal of Medical Imaging and Radiation Sciences, 51*(4), S59–S71.

Taylor, A., Hodgson, D., Gee, M., & Collins, K. (2017). Compassion in healthcare: A concept analysis. *Journal of Radiotherapy in Practice, 16*(4), 350–360.

Walker, M., Quinn, I., & Corder, K. (2016). Improving compassionate care skills with education. *Nursing Times, 112*(17), 21–23.

Weng, H. Y., Lapate, R. C., Stodola, D. E., Rogers, G. M., & Davidson, R. J. (2018). Visual attention to suffering after compassion training is associated with decreased amygdala responses. *Frontiers in Psychology, 9*, 771.

Wilkes, L. M., & Wallis, M. C. (1998). A model of professional nurse caring: Nursing students' experience. *Journal of Advanced Nursing, 27*(3), 582–589. 10.1046/j.1365-2648. 1998.00557.x

# 5

# SELF-CARE

## Introduction

The first of the exercises we will focus on is self-care. It is important to recognise the importance of compassion by starting with ourselves. In this chapter you will learn:

1. What we mean by self-care
2. The opposites of self-care
3. The importance of self-care and why we need it for compassion
4. The obstacles to this strength

## What do we mean by self-care?

Self-care refers to how an individual looks after their well-being. It involves insight, knowledge of self, action to address our own needs, and using a self-soothing kind voice to guide us through. Self-care can take various forms, meaning we need to understand and recognise what works best for us. We are all unique and what might give or deplete energy for one person will differ from another. What gives and takes away our energy can be a small, simple easy fix like skipping breakfast or bigger and complex such as a change in the values we have towards helping. In certain cases, a decline in empathy and compassion for others is often accounted for by the experience of empathy/compassion fatigue and burnout or the everyday grind of work. Working with others who have experienced suffering and trauma is hard. Everyday exposure to the suffering of others, especially in stressful working conditions, can leave us feeling vulnerable and exhausted because of the work we do. Helping is not an easy task and can affect our professional quality of life. While it is perfectly normal to feel this way it can also be a sign for us to engage in self-care activities to support ourselves through the emotional and psychological costs

DOI: 10.4324/9781003276425-5

of working in care, help build resilience, and improve wellbeing. Equally, we can become a victim of our inner critics. The internal bully constantly tells us that we are not good enough or that we are failures. Changing this to a self-compassionate voice that treats us with kindness can help us on our way to self-care and is an important feature when taking a caring and compassionate stance towards our mental health and wellbeing.

It is also important to remember that self-care is not the panacea for alleviating all problems associated with stress in healthcare, and it is not to place the responsibility at the feet of staff. The working environment plays an important part and managers, and leaders must acknowledge this so that both practitioners and compassion can flourish among patients and help foster workplaces where strengths are encouraged, and staff given the space and time to do this. While the exercise set out here is a guide for practitioners to develop self-care techniques, organisations can use these exercises to explore ways in which they can promote wellness in their places of work.

## A focus on self-compassion[1]

Self-compassion has continually been shown to be an effective short-term practice that had long term impact. It can be used as a quick in the moment method of self-care when the stress and strain or work get too much, or when faced with a difficult challenge and a run just is not possible (Even though you might feel like running away). Self-compassion should also be used during the development of your compassion strengths. Learning and progress is never linear. In fact, it is a long and winding road that leads us to where we want to go, and even when we get there, new avenues open and we are once again faced with more decisions. It is in these moments that self-compassion can help us be kinder and gentler to ourselves as we make these important steps forward. It should be there for us when we want to curse the way things are going to remind us of our humanness. We will never really get rid of difficulty, pain, suffering, hurt and disappointment, but with self-compassion with us along the journey we can weather the storm, and take the edge off. So, practice self-compassion whenever things don't seem to be going your way, and it will help soften the blow. Evidence shows that self-compassion mediates self-care, in that when we show kindness to our and suffering, we allow ourselves to feel that pain, but it also motivates us to take care of ourselves too. It can motivate us to eat healthy, exercise, or do things that sustain us because we matter and deserve compassion too. Some themes and exercises will have an underling foundation in self-compassion practices.

## The opposite of self-care

The opposite of self-care is self-neglect where we put ourselves last and everyone and every other thing first. This might seem like a noble endeavour to but the consequences to self and others can be devastating. At its most extreme self-neglect can lead to physical and mental illness. This becomes a paradox of helping. If we do not look after ourselves, how then can we expect to look after others? We might try but eventually, our compassion will become paralysed by stresses and strains. Stress, empathy and compassion fatigue, and burnout are key issues in healthcare that affect the care being provided, resulting in depression, anxiety, and other similar conditions. Healthcare staff have a duty to look after themselves and take the steps necessary to ensure that they can perform their work without risk of harm to themselves and others.

## The importance of self-care and why we need it

In chapter 3, we looked at what hinders compassion and how different working and personal conditions such as a toxic workplace can contribute to feelings of stress, burnout, empathy fatigue, and compassion fatigue. Due to the nature of their work most healthcare practitioners will face these problems in their career. The cause of these things might come from the working environment, the people one works with, or problems at home. Indeed, healthcare practitioners report that barriers in the workplace create more fatigue than compassionate work with patients (Egan et al., 2019). To this end, burnout has been recognised as a medical diagnosis by the World Health Organisation. The symptoms of burnout, vicarious trauma, and compassion fatigue share similarities and can be equally detrimental to practitioners' wellbeing, mental health, and compassion. Burnout correlates with substandard care and low patient satisfaction and more medical errors among nursing and medical staff. Empathy and over-engagement in another suffering can take their toll on our mental health and wellbeing. From the people we work with to the environments we work in, there is an increased risk of burnout, empathy fatigue, vicarious trauma, and compassion fatigue. Self-care is therefore vital for building the resilience needed to perform well at work and live a good life. Our needs are an important aspect of being human that can motivate and help us flourish in work and life. We will not mention work-life balance in this section as it is not about finding balance and more about raising your awareness of your needs and doing what you can to address how you are feeling at any given moment. The key thing about self-care is that it helps replenish our empathy and compassion and helps us flourish in our work and lives.

Self-care activities can be used just for the sake of looking after yourself. In most cases, there are more serious reasons for practicing self-care such as those that are stress-related, for example, compassion fatigue and burnout. Most compassion fatigue and burnout can be addressed early on before it becomes a more severe problem. So that we can act later, in this section I would like you to reflect on what might trigger you or are the warning signs that your mood and wellbeing are being affected. Bur first, to help you identify some of the signs to look out for, here is a list of the common symptoms, risk factors, triggers, and things to re-cognise for yourself and others.

## Obstacles to this strength

There is any number of obstacles that can stand in our way of self-care. They can be self-imposed or imposed on us by the environments we work in. By naming them we can think of ways to overcome these obstacles and tackle that which impedes us with our strengths of compassion. Common reasons are:

*Lack of motivation*
*Self-care is self-indulgent*
*I feel guilty looking after myself*
*I do not have time, or I am too busy*
*It is too late to x (run, go the gym, swim)*
*I do not mediate*
*Self-care is a sign of weakness*
*I have other responsibilities*
*Fears of self-compassion*

What other things get in your way?

_____

_____

_____

_____

_____

While all these are perfectly normal and genuine (I am sure you can think of more) reasons that can prevent you from taking part in a self-care activity, the activities presented here do not have to occupy much of your time and can be worked around a busy schedule. The crucial point to make is that you are doing something that supports your well-being. We can and should take short steps towards self-care. We would not go straight to the gym and expect to lift the heaviest weights or put on our running shoes and run a marathon without any training. It would have the opposite effect on us both mentally and physically. Self-care starts here by acknowledging that and giving yourself a break in the expectations and reasons for why you cannot or should not look after yourself. It also helps to identify what we like and do more of that while trying out new things too. Find time in your day, even if it is moments in the morning or evening either at home or at work to do a little thing. Plan weekly or monthly events in advance around your other commitments so you have something to look forward to but do not feel guilty about.

As we saw in previous chapters, motivation is a key part of learning and developing compassion for self and others. With this in mind, how motivated do you feel on a scale of 1 (not much), to 10 (very much) to engage in self-care activities?

_____

_____

_____

_____

## The evidenced based benefits of self-care for compassion

The need for practitioners to look after themselves is a highly sought-after compassionate quality. Research tells us that stress and burnout result from a lack of self-care. While on the other hand self-care has been shown to aid in building resilience (Rosenberg, 2020). Healthcare practitioners express the need to learn about self-care techniques to sustain themselves, and their compassion and protect themselves from compassion fatigue and burnout (Sinclair et al., 2020). Though self-compassion or mindfulness are effective forms of self-care, individual techniques provide a more comprehensive approach to building resilience, developing emotional strength, and compassion for self and others. Self-care is the things we do for ourselves that are compassionate, while self-compassion is the way we speak and respond to our suffering. Self-compassion can be seen as the heart of self-care and central to the actions we take in times of need to alleviate our suffering. Evidence shows that self-compassion is a significant predictor of both personal and professional self-care among social workers (Miller et al., 2019). To be effective, Mills et al. (2018) propose that self-care should be taken seriously, practitioners should create a plan for what activities will help them, and for leaders to create supportive structures that stimulate these self-care activities in the workplace and at home.

Interventions that encourage self-compassion, mindfulness, and other spiritual pursuits have shown promising results for both healthcare students and practitioners with burnout and compassion fatigue (Beaumont et al., 2017; Duarte et al., 2016; Mathad et al., 2017). For example, student practitioners who are kinder to themselves are more likely to experience compassion satisfaction, be compassionate to others, and less likely to be burned out by their work, than those who criticise themselves harshly. Self-compassion helps individuals to recognise their own suffering and motivates them to protect themselves during tough times. Other approaches to self-care that reduce stress and burnout include physical, emotional, cognitive/mental, spiritual, and social strategies. The most effective of these include spending time with family and friends, prayer, yoga, physical exercise, affirmations, and hobbies (Kravits et al., 2010). These practices help us become aware of our own needs and suffering, and with this awareness, we inadvertently become more attuned to the suffering of the people we support and treat in our work. Self-care can help increase overall compassion for others, improve wellbeing, and decrease burnout over time too. Learning about these techniques and finding out which ones work best are key for developing your compassion strengths (Durkin et al., 2022).

## Types of self-care

Self-care is more than making sure you get a good night's sleep or hitting the gym every night, it is about taking a holistic look at your overall health and wellbeing and looking after your physical, emotional, spiritual, social, professional, and psychological needs. There is a complete range of different self-care activities and exercises that fall into six categories that can be performed to alleviate stress, and low mood, and to improve wellbeing.

## Physical

Physical self-care is about how much sleep you get, the foods you eat, the exercise you do, and how much you put into looking after your overall physical health. These types of activities use all your body and get you moving. It is important to remember that our body and mind are connected. A healthy body equates to a healthy mind and vice versa.

---

**BOX 5.1   SELF-CARE**

Ask yourself:

*Am I getting enough quality sleep?*
*Am I exercising regularly?*
*Am I eating healthy foods that nourish me?*

---

Dance, Move, Healthy eating habits, sleep regularly, engage in activity/hobbies, Exercise, Medical care when needed, Preventative medical care, take time to be sexual with self or partner, take time off from work, and take a holiday. Exercise such as running, walking, or type of physical activity will not end your stress, but it will help you manage it. Exercise is a fantastic way to clear your mind, reduce the intensity of the emotions you might be feeling, and help you see with more clarity what is affecting you so that you can manage your problems and return to your compassionate self. You could go for a walk or run in the park or in the countryside. Aim to get out as often as possible. You can do this on your own, or with other people and dogs if you have them.

## Emotional

Emotional self-care concerns the practices that serve our emotional needs and allow us to acknowledge and express our feelings in helpful ways. Talking to a trusted friend, supervisor, colleague, or someone you trust about your feelings, or another activity enables you to process and release any uncomfortable emotions associated with stress such as anxiety, depression, frustration, and anger in healthy ways. It is helpful to have strategies in place that can help you manage these emotions and build a tolerance to distress.

---

### BOX 5.2 EMOTIONAL

Things to ask yourself:

*Do you engage in activities that energise and replenish you?*
*What do you do with uncomfortable emotions?*
*How do you speak to your emotional self?*

---

You can focus on things like self-compassion, self-soothing talk, and doing something to boost your mood. Take part in a positive activity, laugh, play, spend time with people you enjoy, play with your children, or give yourself praise. You can allow yourself to cry. You can re-watch a favourite movie(s) or re-read a favourite book(s). Self-compassion is a terrific way to develop compassion for others and improve your well-being. Studies show how self-compassion can alleviate our suffering, compassion fatigue, and our negative inner critic, and improve well-being and compassion for others. Getting to the root of our pain and treating those parts that need it most with kindness and compassion can make a real difference to our wellbeing. Self-compassion will feature throughout this book with suggestions from various compassion researchers and practitioners.

## Spiritual

Research shows that having faith in something bigger than yourself whether that be God or the universe, can help foster resilience and reduce stress. Developing a deeper sense of meaning with and connection to the world around you, either through meditation, prayer, or being in nature is good for the soul and lead a healthy life. Exercises like gratitude can keep us grounded, and thankful for what we have, build hope, and make us optimistic for the future.

---

### BOX 5.3 SPIRITUAL

Things to ask yourself:

*What are you doing to nourish your soul?*
*Are you engaging in activities that fulfil you at a spiritual level?*

---

You might meditate, go to a place of worship, practice gratitude, or connect to nature. You can visualise yourself having a positive day, or you could sing. Read inspirational or practice yoga. The stoics had a phrase that relates to extreme gratitude, "Amori Fati", which roughly translates as "love of fate". This means that no matter what happens to you, good or bad, say to yourself "I am grateful for this" because it is helping me in one way or another.

## Simple exercise - gratitude

A simple thing you can do each day to help your well-being is to look for the positive in your life, and express gratitude for them. Attending to thoughts of what we don't have leaves us in a negative state. Apricating what we have can do wonders for your well-being and help you create a positive outlook. Be grateful for the small things too. Research shows that this can have a greater effect on your wellbeing and happiness (Wood et al., 2010).

Write down six things (or more) big or small that you are grateful for

1. _____
2. _____
3. _____
4. _____
5. _____
6. _____

## Social

Humans are social beings meaning we need to be around and connect with others. Building and maintaining relationships is a terrific way to connect to others that can help you flourish and is critical for your wellbeing. It can be hard sometimes to find time for others, especially with competing work demands and bust lives. However, figuring out a schedule that serves both you and your friends and family can bring benefits to your self-care.

---

**BOX 5.4   SOCIAL**

Things to ask yourself:

*Are you spending enough quality time with your friends and family?*
*What activities do you engage in that support your health and wellbeing?*

---

Connect with family and friends. Spending time with people that nourish you. Set a date for either your significant other or a friend. Depending on the relationship make it romantic and special in a way that fits. Do something fun together. Connect with someone you have not spoken to in a while. Also, think about the people in your life that drains your energy, think about limiting your time with them or cutting them out completely.

## Professional

We spend the most of our day at work. It is therefore important that we take steps to ensure that our place of work and the people in it do not have too much of a negative impact on our wellbeing. We can end up working longer hours, extra shifts, or taking on more than we can manage. These all take their toll on us sometime, leading to burnout and stress, which affects our ability to show compassion. There are things you can do to put things in place that create a healthy environment for your mind and yourself.

---

**BOX 5.5  PROFESSIONAL**

Ask yourself:

*How is my work affecting my mental health and wellbeing?*
*Am I doing enough to create boundaries and limit my responsibilities to a manageable workload?*

---

Take time to chat with co-workers. Set limits with patients/clients/service users. Take breaks during the workday. Discuss cases with colleagues. Make quiet time to complete tasks. Arrange your workspace so it is comforting. Get regular supervision, (if possible). Diversify your caseload. Participate in professional education/training, take part in (or set up) a peer support group. Negotiate your needs. Set reminders for regular breaks and take them. Take a different route home from work, even if it takes a little longer, and make it one that is scenic and less stressful than traffic. Speak to your manager about how you are feeling.

## Psychological

Attending to your psychological needs includes activities that keep you mentally healthy. Our minds can become a place of pain and distress, especially when under pressure from work-related or personal issues. We can become self-critical, judging, and our worst enemy. Developing awareness and self-compassion for ourselves can help change our self-talk to a more positive and healthier inner dialogue.

There are other activities that you can do such as reading or watching something that stimulates your mind in an effective way.

---

### BOX 5.6 PSYCHOLOGICAL

Ask yourself:

*Are you spending enough time doing things that mentally stimulate you?*
*How do you speak to yourself, particularly when you are under stress?*

---

To develop this, you can practice being mindful, or reading non-work-related literature. You could even take time out of your day for reflection. Maybe setting goals for yourself would help. Say "no" to extra activities. Develop a plan for caring for yourself. Participate in your therapy or write in a journal. Use positive self-talk. Unplug from the world, switch off your phone and be alone with yourself. Build hope and optimism by thinking about what you want for your future and how you might get there.

## Summary

### Definition

Self-care is defined as *"the practice of taking an active role in protecting one's well-being and happiness, in particular during periods of stress."* As a strength of compassion, it is the things we do for ourselves that enable us to be compassionate.

### Key indicators

Self-compassion, Resilience, Exercise, Spiritual pursuits, Emotional strength, Resilience, Looking after self, Mediation, Exercise.

### Psychology

Self-care covers our emotional, cognitive, and behaviour psychology in that we can do things that boost our wellbeing, say kind thoughts to ourselves when we are struggling, and do things that nourish our emotions in positive ways.

### Evidenced by

Engages in self-care practices that help reduce stress and increase compassion. Examples include healthy eating, exercise, yoga, mindfulness, self-compassion, and socialising.

## Prevalence of that strength

Self-care can help students and practitioners show compassion for others and improve mental wellbeing. It is a highly sought-after strength of a compassionate practitioner. Self-care is strongly related to overall compassion strengths.

## Reflective questions

*What am I currently doing or can do to show this strength in myself (and others)?*
*Is self-care selfish or necessary for my development and compassion?*
*Does self-care help me become more resilient?*

## Combing strengths

**Self-care** goes well with **empathy, communication, and connection**, in that it helps raise our awareness of needs, we can communicate to ourselves how we are feeling, empathise with that feeling, recognise and connect to what we need, and treat ourselves with compassion and care.

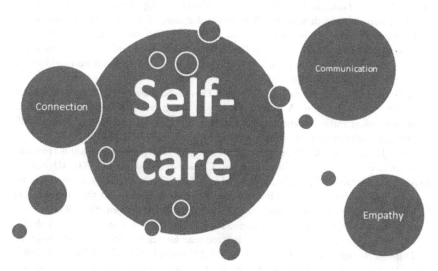

**FIGURE 5.1** How self-care combines with other compassion strengths

## Conclusion

In this chapter, we have explored what self-care is, what it is not, why it is important, the different types of self-care, and how to recognise our needs. Using the REPS method, you will be able to build this compassion strength and develop a working plan that you can use to bring more compassionate thought and action into your own life and practice. Incorporate this strength into your everyday life and practice and combine this strength with the others in ways that bring the benefits of compassion to both you and your patients.

What have you learned that you did not know before?

_____

_____

_____

_____

_____

## Note

1 https://self-compassion.org

## References

Beaumont, E., Rayner, G., Durkin, M., & Bowling, G. (2017). The effects of Compassionate Mind Training on student psychotherapists. *The Journal of Mental Health Training, Education and Practice, 12*(5), 300–312.

Duarte, J., Pinto-Gouveia, J., & Cruz, B. (2016). Relationships between nurses' empathy, self-compassion and dimensions of professional quality of life: A cross-sectional study. *International Journal of Nursing Studies, 60*, 1–11. 10.1016/j.ijnurstu.2016.02.015

Durkin, M., Gurbutt, R., & Carson, J. (2022). Effectiveness of an online short compassion strengths course on nursing students compassion: A mixed methods non-randomised pilot study. *Nurse Education Today, 111*, 105315.

Egan, H., Keyte, R., McGowan, K., Peters, L., Lemon, N., Parsons, S., … & Mantzios, M. (2019). 'You before me': A qualitative study of health care professionals' and students' understanding and experiences of compassion in the workplace, self-compassion, self-care and health behaviours. *Health Professions Education, 5*(3), 225–236.

Jay Miller, J., Lee, J., Niu, C., Grise-Owens, E., & Bode, M. (2019). Self-compassion as a predictor of self-care: A study of social work clinicians. *Clinical Social Work Journal, 47*(4), 321–331.

Kravits, K., McAllister-Black, R., Grant, M., & Kirk, C. (2010). Self-care strategies for nurses: A psycho-educational intervention for stress reduction and the prevention of burnout. *Applied Nursing Research, 23*(3), 130–138. 10.1016/j.apnr.2008.08.002

Mathad, M. D., Pradhan, B., & Sasidharan, R. K. (2017). Effect of yoga on psychological functioning of nursing students: A randomized wait list control trial. *Journal of Clinical and Diagnostic Research: JCDR, 11*(5), KC01–KC05. 10.7860%2FJCDR%2F2017%2F26517.9833

Mills, J., Wand, T., & Fraser, J. A. (2018). Examining self-care, self-compassion and compassion for others: a cross-sectional survey of palliative care nurses and doctors. *International Journal of Palliative Nursing, 24*(1), 4–11.

Rosenberg, Abby R. (2020). Cultivating Deliberate Resilience During the Coronavirus Disease 2019 Pandemic. *JAMA Pediatrics, 174*, 817–818. 10.1001/jamapediatrics.2020.1436.

Sinclair, Shane, Kondejewski, Jane, Schulte, Fiona, Letourneau, Nicole, Kuhn, Susan, Raffin-Bouchal, Shelley, Guilcher, Gregory M.T., & Strother, Douglas (2020). Compassion in Pediatric Healthcare: A Scoping Review. *Journal of Pediatric Nursing, 51*, 57–6610.1016/j.pedn.2019.12.009.

Wood, A. M., Froh, J. J., & Geraghty, A. W. (2010). Gratitude and well-being: A review and theoretical integration. *Clinical psychology review, 30*(7), 890–905. 10.1016/j.cpr.2010.03.005

# 6

# EMPATHY

## Introduction

The second exercise is about developing the strength of empathy. Empathy is a vital part and strength of compassion. It links with other strengths such as connection, interpersonal skills, and communication to help us understand others and what they are experiencing in their time of need. In this chapter you will learn:

1. What we mean by empathy
2. The opposites of empathy
3. Why we need it in healthcare
4. The obstacles to this empathy
5. The types of empathy

## What is empathy?

Empathy is the way we use our thoughts and feelings to understand another. You might have heard of it being referred to as putting yourself in someone else's shoes or seeing things from the other person's perspective. The term empathy comes from the German word "*Einfühlung*," which means "feeling-in." It was the psychologist Titchener (1867–1927) who translated it into English. The Dutch words 'midglide' or 'meelijden' which means "feeling the same" are also used to describe empathy. Empathy is associated with the theory of mind, in that we can reason what others are going through (Vollm et al., 2006). The psychologist, Carl Rogers (1957) defined empathy as "the capability to sense the client's private world as if it were your own". Another defines empathic listening as "the ability to enter into and understand the world of another person and to communicate this understanding of them" (Egan, 1990). Quite often empathy is associated with the understanding of emotions,

DOI: 10.4324/9781003276425-6

however Davis (1983) views it as a multidimensional construct consisting of perspective taking, fantasy, empathic concern, and personal distress. For example, with empathic concern, "we feel upset" because "they feel upset." This may lead the practitioner to avoid the patient because of the personal distress they feel being with this person. For instance, Bloom (2017), argues that cognitive empathy has a more protective factor than emotional empathy as the latter leads to burnout and is not the best use of our empathic resources because it makes us vulnerable to the feelings of another. In this respect, Sinclair et al., (2017) propose that emotional empathy has a potentially darker side, in that it can cause burnout in the caregiver. Thus, with perspective taking, you can rationalise how someone might feel based on what they are going through, make predictions about the causes of their behaviour, and limit the risk of empathic distress. The ability to understand another's perspective is associated with greater compassion and lower personal distress (Davis, 2018). This is not to dismiss emotional empathy because this reaction is out of our control, but to see that there are different approaches to empathy. Overall, empathy is the motivation to understand another's situation that requires emotional and cognitive skills that can inspire compassion. It is much more than putting yourself in someone else's shoes. Empathy is about understanding what it feels like, what it is like, to walk in those shoes for the person wearing them and acknowledge and validate their experiences.

## The opposite of empathy

The opposite of empathy is apathy, but egocentricity can also be an oppositive too. Apathy is defined as the lack of interest in others, or the motivation to care about what is happening around you. With apathy, you lack the desire to see things from the other's perspective and do not feel what someone is feeling. You can feel little enthusiasm or concern for others. It can affect your work and be a result of burnout. Equally, egocentricity is when one thinks more about themself than others. In healthcare, it can be the practitioner who believes more in their ability than the considerations of someone else's.

## Why do we need empathy?

From an evolutionary perspective knowing that someone else was in danger helped when making the judgement if that threat extended to us. Empathy is recognised globally as being fundamental to compassionate care, and therapeutic relationships (Moudatsou et al., 2020). Through the power of understanding, unconditional positive regard, empathy has the power to open doors and overcome blocks to healing (Rogers, 1957). Studies into perspective taking reveal positive outcomes for empathy. For example, when cognitive empathy, such as perspective taking is used practitioners experience greater job satisfaction, work engagement, and retention, while the opposite happens for emotional empathy (Dal Santo et al., 2014). Oppositive to that, too much emotional empathy can make use more susceptible to burnout and empathy fatigue. Intrinsically, practitioners can adapt their emotional empathy to include more perspective taking. Empathy is associated with reductions in pain, increased practitioner well-being, and improved patient care and satisfaction (Howick & Rees, 2017). It can be effective for patients when showing their symptoms. For example, patients are more open about their condition when they note their physicians responding with empathy to their verbal cues (Finset & Ørnes, 2017), and are more closed off when it is not shown (Halpern 2007). Empathy helps connect patient and practitioner on a deeper level and is the bridge between seeing into the core of a person and their suffering. A greater therapeutic alliance is achieved between client and therapist when the therapist's empathy is higher (Malin & Pos, 2015). Empathy is expressed through the cognitive or emotional aspects of thought and feeling, rather than the expressed behaviour one might see with compassion. As we saw in earlier chapters, empathy can be challenging. Seeing what the other sees and what they feel is not always easy. For instance, being with someone who has been through challenging times and suffered immensely, can trigger deep emotions in us. Equally, a student or practitioner may feel less empathy for a patient who is considered 'difficult,' because of the demands they make without considering what lies behind their behaviour. If a patient who has been convicted of a crime against another human may be viewed as deserving of their suffering and not of compassion. In contrast, driven by a compassionate response, concern for the patient's experiences, regardless of the crime, might help practitioners see these patients with more understanding. While this is not always easy, it is necessary. Learning to manage these deep-seated emotions can aid you in managing them as you care for the person. On the other hand, perspective taking which is where we use our rational mind to understand another's suffering is seen as a more practical response to suffering. Where emotional empathy is seen as being out of the control of the practitioner, perspective taking is considered a deliberate process (Stansfield et al., 2016). This approach reduces the emotional aspect of compassion which can potentially lead to burnout. It also makes us focus our attention on the individual. Although in certain professions this is necessary, sometimes there is more than one person who needs empathy. Despite this knowledge, it is not always that easy to avoid feeling another's suffering. Equally, this line of thinking does not take into consideration how thoughts and feelings are intertwined. Some people think that due to its emotional content empathy cannot be controlled and tend to see its benefits through a narrow view. As a result, they are less likely to embrace challenges associated with attending to the emotional needs of others (Zaki, 2017). Even though there are arguments for both cognitive and affective empathy studies suggest that healthcare workers with higher emotional empathy are more likely to sanitise their hands when reminded that it helps their patients (Grant & Hofmann, 2011).

## Obstacles to empathy

What obstacles might get in your way of expressing empathy? How about someone who annoys us, a patient or colleague for example? The wonderful thing about empathy is that we don't have to like that person to understand them. We can look beyond the presenting behaviours and see what it might be that is causing them to be how they are in that present moment. Although easy to empathise with the victim of abuse, it would be exceedingly difficult to show empathy or feel with an abuser. What about the drug abuser? We might judge them for not being deserving. Or a homeless person asking for money. We might want to through empathy but fear of them using that money to buy drugs or alcohol may prevent us from doing. This limits our ability to show compassion and care for others. Empathy helps us understand what they need, and what we can do for them. Others may be:

*Struggling to see things from another perspective*
*Burned out*
*Judgements*
*Not listening or being fully present*
*Feeling helpless*
*The pain of feeling another suffering*
*being stuck in your head*
*Distractions*
*Self-esteem*

What other things get in your way?

_____
_____
_____
_____
_____

How motivated do you feel on a scale of 1 (not much), to 10 (very much) to engage in empathy?

_____
_____
_____
_____
_____

## Simple exercise – a compassion strengths approach to empathy fatigue

Sometime when working with people who experience difficult emotions such as fear, distress and anger it can feel as though these emotions are our own. Empathy has the power to connect us to others but in doing so it also leaves us vulnerable to their suffering. The pain we feel from this can make us want to run or shut off (fight or flight) from them, which then leaves us stressed, tired and unable to do our best.

A simple exercise to help you with working with emotions that arise from being empathic, is to connect to that part of you that is hurting and bring to your awareness the emotion you are feeling. Resisting will only make the feeling worse, whereas acknowledge how you feel will give you ownership of your experience, and the impact it is having on you. Once you have identified this, using compassionate communication you can verbalise what you are feeling, and use soothing compassionate tones to develop kindness and acceptance towards yourself.

## The evidenced based benefits of empathy for compassion

As discussed in the earlier chapter, empathy is often mistaken for compassion. The difference is that compassion takes empathy to the next stage and does something to address the feelings and suffering that the other person is experiencing. In this way, empathy is the predictor of compassionate action. As Figley (2002) states compassion needs deep empathy towards suffering for it to be realised. Empathy is the important first step that practitioners make so the person they are with feels heard, understood, validated, and listened to. Without this ability to feel or understand the inner states of patients and clients, practitioners cannot be compassionate. Research highlights the importance of empathy and its connection to compassion (Kneasfey et al., 2015). In the UK, empathy is key to compassionate practice. Empathy enables the practitioner to be emotionally moved by another's suffering and is what helps motivate them to alleviate it (Gustin & Wagner, 2013). When helping others, empathy can lead to feelings of well-being and reinforce kindness. Empathy is the key to understanding the thoughts and feelings of others. Empathy drives the practitioner toward this understanding and is key to them demonstrating compassion for others (Gerace & Rigney, 2020). Although we can never fully know what someone feels inside, empathy can give us a peek into another's internal world and help us understand them and feel understood. Practitioners can follow up with other compassionate behaviours and actions making use of these strengths to aid in the alleviation of distress and suffering.

## Types of empathy

As we saw in the chapter about what hinders compassion, there is a risk of empathy fatigue or empathic distress occurring when empathising with our patients. There are several types of empathy though, and each can have a different outcome. Empathy, like compassion, is multifaceted. It is emotional as well as cognitive. Both are helpful, while one may create problems or opportunities depending on how we look at it. We shall explore some of the different kinds.

## Emotional empathy

Emotional empathy covers a multitude of ways in which this type of empathy can be expressed. For example, feeling with, experience sharing, personal distress, or having an affective part. Emotional empathy has a biological element to it in that experiencing another's emotions leads to concern for the other, in that seeing another's suffering stirs up feelings in us. This can help us communicate what they are going through using feelings to support this.

---

**BOX 6.1 EMOTIONAL EMPATHY**

Ask yourself:

*Am I moved emotionally by the person's story?*
*Do I feel what they are feeling?*

---

Imagine what it feels to be that person, understand, and validate their feelings. It can help to name their feelings and show acceptance of what emotions they express. Make a statement that shows that you recognise their experience and the feelings attached to their experiences. Encourage the person to talk about how they are feeling and be open to receiving what they say. For example, "*It can help me understand what you are going through and how this is affecting you emotionally.*"

## Cognitive empathy

As the name suggests cognitive empathy includes a cognitive component. We use cognitive representations to detect and recognise the emotional states of others based on their expressions and stories. It is also described as mentalizing or perspective taking, in that we can perceive what another is feeling without having to experience what they are feeling.

---

**BOX 6.2 COGNITIVE EMPATHY**

Ask yourself:

*Can I imagine what it is like to be this person?*
*Am I able to rationalise that their experience has not been good for them?*

---

Imagine what they must be going through, the thoughts that are running through their mind, and all their worries. Understanding what it must be like to be in their position can help you show understanding of their problems. Validate their experience. Seeing that what is happening is a very authentic experience for them. For example, "*I can see how you would feel that way considering what you are/have been through.*"

Use positive praise for showing courage and progress, no matter how small. For example, "*it must have taken a lot of bravery to tell me that just now.*"

## Summary

### Definition

Empathy can be defined as the ability to sense another's emotions and understand things from their perspective and share that back with them.

### Key indicators

The perspective of the patient, putting self in the patient's shoes, Feeling the patient's suffering.

### Psychology

The psychologies present in empathy are emotional and cognitive as these are the two primary means of understanding the thoughts and feelings of others.

### Evidenced by

Deeper consideration of the patient's situation to get a greater understanding of what they are experiencing. Acting in a way that you would like to be treated or someone close to you.

### Prevalence of this strength

Empathy is considered a vital strength by those who work in healthcare. It is the gateway to understanding and can be combined with other strengths to enable understanding and action.

### Reflective questions

*What am I currently doing or can do to show this strength in myself (and others)?*
*If I do not have empathy, can I still demonstrate compassion for others?*
*Which empathy do I use, affective or perspective taking, or both?*

### Combing strengths

**Empathy** combines well with **interpersonal skills, communication, and connection,** in that it helps raise our awareness of needs, we can communicate to ourselves how we are feeling, empathise with that feeling, recognise and connect to what we need, and treat ourselves with compassion and care.

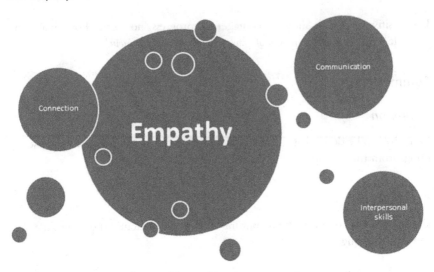

**FIGURE 6.1** How empathy combines with other compassion strengths

## Conclusion

This chapter has been about empathy. While empathy and compassion are often confused for one another, it is important to remember how different they are. Another key factor with empathy is the different types and how they can both lead to different conclusions and results for the practitioner. Being aware of the impact of emotional empathy can help you decide which type to use and in what situation.

What have you learned that you did not know before?

_____
_____
_____
_____
_____

## References

Bloom, P. (2017). *Against empathy: The case for rational compassion.* London: Random House.

Dal Santo, L., Pohl, S., Saiani, L., & Battistelli, A. (2014). Empathy in the emotional interactions with patients. Is it positive for nurses too?. *Journal of Nursing Education and Practice, 4*(2), 74.

Davis, A. C., Leppanen, W., Mularczyk, K. P., Bedard, T., & Stroink, M. L. (2018). Systems thinkers express an elevated capacity for the allocentric components of cognitive and affective empathy. *Systems Research and Behavioral Science, 35*(2), 216–229.

Davis, M. H. (1983). Measuring individual differences in empathy: Evidence for a multidimensional approach. *Journal of Personality and Social Psychology, 44*(1), 113–126. 10.1037/0022-3514.44.1.113

Egan, G. (1990). *The skilled helper: A systematic approach to effective helping.* Thomson Brooks/ Cole Publishing Co.

Figley, C. R. (2002). Compassion fatigue: Psychotherapists' chronic lack of self care. *Journal of clinical psychology, 58*(11), 1433–1441.

Finset, A., & Ørnes, K. (2017). Empathy in the clinician–patient relationship: the role of reciprocal adjustments and processes of synchrony. *Journal of patient experience, 4*(2), 64–68.

Gerace, A., & Rigney, G. (2020). Considering the relationship between sleep and empathy and compassion in mental health nurses: It's time. *International Journal of Mental Health Nursing, 29*(5), 1002–1010.

Grant, A. M., & Hofmann, D. A. (2011). It's not all about me: Motivating hand hygiene among health care professionals by focusing on patients. *Psychological science, 22*(12), 1494–1499.

Halpern, J. (2007). Empathy and patient–physician conflicts. *Journal of general internal medicine, 22*(5), 696–700.

Howick, J., & Rees, S. (2017). Overthrowing barriers to empathy in healthcare: empathy in the age of the Internet. *Journal of the Royal Society of Medicine, 110*(9), 352–357.

Kneafsey, R., Brown, S., Sein, K., Chamley, C., & Parsons, J. (2015). A qualitative study of key stakeholders' perspectives on compassion in healthcare and the development of a framework for compassionate interpersonal relations. *Journal of Clinical Nursing, 25,* 70–79. 10.1111/jocn.12964

Malin, A. J., & Pos, A. E. (2015). The impact of early empathy on alliance building, emotional processing, and outcome during experiential treatment of depression. *Psychotherapy Research, 25*(4), 445–459.

Moudatsou, M., Stavropoulou, A., Philalithis, A., & Koukouli, S. (2020, January). The role of empathy in health and social care professionals. In *Healthcare* (Vol. 8, No. 1, p. 26). MDPI.

Rogers, C. R. (1957). The necessary and sufficient conditions of therapeutic personality change. *Journal of Consulting Psychology, 21*(2), 95–103. 10.1037/h0045357

Sinclair, S., Beamer, K., Hack, T. F., McClement, S., Raffin Bouchal, S., Chochinov, H. M., & Hagen, N. A. (2017). Sympathy, empathy, and compassion: A grounded theory study of palliative care patients' understandings, experiences, and preferences. *Palliative medicine, 31*(5), 437–447.

Stansfield, R. Brent, Schwartz, Alan, O'Brien, Celia Laird, Dekhtyar, Michael, Dunham, Lisette, & Quirk, Mark (2015). Development of a metacognitive effort construct of empathy during clinical training: a longitudinal study of the factor structure of the Jefferson Scale of Empathy. *Advances in Health Sciences Education, 21,* 5–17. 10.1007/ s10459-015-9605-1.

Völlm, Birgit A., Taylor, Alexander N.W., Richardson, Paul, Corcoran, Rhiannon, Stirling, John, McKie, Shane, Deakin, John F.W., & Elliott, Rebecca (2006). Neuronal correlates of theory of mind and empathy: A functional magnetic resonance imaging study in a nonverbal task. *NeuroImage, 29,* 90–98. 10.1016/j.neuroimage.2005.07.022.

Wiklund Gustin, L., & Wagner, L. (2013). The butterfly effect of caring–clinical nursing teachers' understanding of self-compassion as a source to compassionate care. *Scandinavian Journal of Caring Sciences, 27*(1), 175–183.

Zaki, J. (2017). Moving beyond stereotypes of empathy. *Trends in Cognitive Sciences, 21*(2), 59–60. 10.1016/j.tics.2016.12.004

# 7

# COMPASSIONATE COMMUNICATION

## Introduction

Compassionate communication is another key element of compassion. It is the way we express ourselves using words, our body language, and listening skills to express compassion to others. In this chapter you will learn:

1. What we mean by communication
2. The opposites of communication
3. The importance of effective communication
4. The obstacles to this strength
5. The types of communication and you might express them

## What is compassionate communication?

Communication is the way people express themselves and exchange information through words, body language, or listening. Communication is done on a one-to-one basis or in groups. It is usually done in person but now with more access to technologies that enable this, there are increased ways of communicating remotely. This means someone can speak to another person anywhere in the world. This great advance brings benefits but at the same time problems. As we rely on other social cues when communicating that digital technology does not provide, yet. In the future, we will see this. Communication in a healthcare setting is quite different from everyday communication. It involves verbal, non-verbal, tone, and active listening. Communication is key to all human and non-human interactions. From the day we are born we communicate our wants and needs making it fundamental for our survival. It is how we share and develop ideas, and express our points of view, desires, dreams, and feelings. It is used to reach an agreement and

DOI: 10.4324/9781003276425-7

develop a mutual understanding with others. Communication is a skill that can influence our own as well as others' lives.

## The opposite of compassionate communication

Because we want communication to be effective, the opposite of effective communication is poor communication. Poor communication can lead to complications in healthcare. Misdiagnosis is common. Feeling that they are not being listened to can create a breakdown in the therapeutic alliance between the patient and practitioner and effectively shut down any chance of progress. Being closed off with your body language can make others feel uncomfortable and that you are not interested or approachable. Similarly, interrupting people when they are talking or rushing them to finish, are obvious signs of poor and ineffective compassionate communication. They send the message to the patient that they are not important, or worthy of your time. This then leads to a breakdown in communication and prevents the delivery of truly compassionate care.

## The importance of compassionate communication in healthcare

In healthcare effective compassionate communication helps the patient or client feel understood and the practitioner understand what to do to improve wellbeing. It is expressed through the language of care, being helpful, giving, supportiveness, and understanding (Crawford et al., 2013). The ability to communicate in a manner that is both professional and personable is encouraged among healthcare students and practitioners in all disciplines around the world. Patients and clients not only want the facts, but they also want this information to be delivered in a caring and compassionate manner. Compassionate communication is an initiative-taking communication style that can help students and practitioners recognise when they are reacting to or engaging in compassion, which in turn improves the understanding and care shown to patients. It is how caregivers make effective use of their listening skills, and not just talk to patients. They listen with the whole body by showing understanding of patients' experiences, through non-verbal expression, and tone of voice. It involves listening attentively to patients, especially when attending to sensitive issues, and making beneficial use of compassionate conversations. Both students and professionals can learn how to ask patients the questions that allow for their story to be told, their suffering confirmed, and their needs met, without first automatically assuming they knew what was going on. Learning how to communicate with compassion is a valuable commodity that can be taught. Now more than ever due to the restrictions imposed on practitioners because of Covid-19, it is important to develop effective communication that is compassionate. Whether it is in person or virtual, having the skills and ability to express compassion to patients and clients makes the difference in how they respond to care, get the help, and support they need. Effective compassionate communication goes beyond clinical knowledge and ability. It enables practitioners to reach those they care for on a personal level. When you think about it, this makes sense. Remember a time when you have been listened to and spoken to with compassion and compare that to a time when you have not. I'm sure you will know the difference straight away.

As a healthcare practitioner, it is a privilege to be able to advocate for the safety of patients. Visiting a practitioner or therapist can be a worrying and daunting experience. Therefore, communicating effectively is a vital skill that helps empower patients to express how they are feeling and show their needs so that they can be supported in a way that is unique to them. Using effective compassionate communication can enable them to feel safe enough to disclose sensitive information. Effective communication can help build trust and express understanding between patients and practitioners. As a result, patients feel more secure. This helps them speak about their needs, worries, and wants, while the practitioner gains valuable insight into what these needs are and explores ways to meet them with the patient. Empowering the patient in this way means that they can take control of their care independently from the care provider. A lack of compassionate communication can be detrimental to the care provided. For example, one of the leading causes of hospital deaths is communication errors, double the errors due to inadequate clinical skills (Coiera, 2006).

## Obstacles to this strength

The costs and benefits of communication can help motivate you toward achieving your development goals. Numerous barriers can get in the way of effective compassionate communication and becoming more aware of them can help practitioners find what might be holding them back.

*Language barriers*
*Lack of insight*
*No training*
*Limited understanding of the diagnosis*
*Neglect of non-verbal cues*
*Masks*
*Distress and emotions*
*Learning difficulties*
*Sensory impairments*
*Jargon*
*Indifference*
*Distractions*
*Dismissiveness*
*Personality*
*Bad mood*

What other things get in your way?

_____

_____

_____

_____

_____

How motivated do you feel on a scale of 1 (not much), to 10 (very much) to communicate compassionately with self and others?

Self: _____

Others: _____

## The evidenced based benefits of communication for compassionate practice

Communication is vital for fostering positive relationships as it helps connect the practitioner and the patient. Compassionate communication is about adapting the skills of communication to the definition of compassion, such as expressing verbal and non-verbal awareness of suffering, coupled with words that convey motivation to alleviate the suffering and meet the needs of the client.

As a result, communication between staff, patients, and their families is viewed as compassionate Bramley and Matiti (2014). Having good listening skills and using a suitable tone of voice, is especially beneficial when breaking bad or sensitive news. Actively listening to patients is highly valued to show compassion. Having emotional communication skills such as listening carefully, encouraging expression, having warm conversations, and expressing interest help people open up. Listening is equally as crucial for compassionate care, as it allows patients to tell their stories (Van der Cingel, 2011). Appreciative caring conversations with patients are effective ways to express compassion through communication (Dewar & Nolan, 2013). Opening a dialogue, using supportive words, really listening and tone of voice are considered compassionate by patients (Sinclair et al., 2016). Communication embraces both verbal and non-verbal exchanges between patient and practitioner is key to compassionate care. Non-verbal communication such as offering a warm smile, demeanour posture, and eye contact are all expressions of compassion. Effective use of body language can also be used to communicate an understanding of the patient's needs (Tehranineshat et al., 2018). Collectively these abilities make practitioners more approachable. Open honest communication can give patients and clients hope. Compassionate communication involves acknowledging another's suffering, expressing care, and understanding, not judging that person or their experience, and putting their needs first. It goes beyond the regular types of communication such as active listening and building rapport and includes communicating sensitively, as well as addressing emotional and existential needs. It also requires the practitioner to communicate their support and understanding of the client/patient and check in with them that they are being treated with compassion (Sinclair et al., 2020) and involves listening for meaning (Way & Tracy, 2012).

## Types of communication

There are ways in which we can communicate effectively with others. They fall into four main categories: verbal, non-verbal (body language), para-verbal (tone, pitch, volume), and active listening. Did you know that when communicating with others, most deal with the verbal content even though that constitutes only 10% of the message, and that non-verbal and para verbal make up the other 90%? We will look at this in more detail now with examples of how each type can be expressed.

## Verbal communication

A considerable proportion of our communication is done through the words we speak. Most people would consider themselves competent speakers and can sometimes feel offended when asked to learn or develop their verbal communication skills. Yet, communication difficulties can lead to complaints from patients and less effective care due to misunderstandings. Verbal communication is used in a variety of ways and settings. For example, when breaking difficult news, or when speaking to patients at the bedside. Effective verbal communication involves listening, pauses, and responses to the other person, and helps foster a two-way dialogue between you and the other person.

---

**BOX 7.1   VERBAL COMMUNICATION**

Things to ask yourself:

*Do I deliver news, and speak compassionately?*
*How am I speaking to patients and clients?*

---

A remarkably simple yet effective mode of compassionate communication is to say hello and introduce yourself. Asking open questions (Socratic), Inquiring, introducing, language barriers, encouraging expression, giving your name, and asking how they would like to be referred, use encouraging words and positive compassionate language. Consider your client/patient. What is their language? How can you compassionately speak to them? Clarifying that they have heard what you have said by asking them can ensure that they feel understood. You might ask:

> *What is your name?*
> *Tell me what is going to tell me about your pain/suffering/situation?*
> *How are you feeling?*
> *What would you like to talk about?*

*How long have you felt like this?*
*I'm sorry you feel that way*
*It must be difficult ....*
*Asking if the client or patient feels they are being treated with compassion*
*You are doing well!*
*I'm not sure about that but I will find out.*
*When you asked about x (therapy/medicine/treatment), was there a particular x you*
*wanted to know more about?*

## Para verbal (tone, pitch, volume, speed)

Given that 10% is verbal, and 70% is non-verbal, 20% is paraverbal and dependent on how the message is delivered. Not only the words we use but the way we convey the message or how it is received can affect the patient.

---

### BOX 7.2   PARA VERBAL

Things to ask yourself:

*How do I ask questions?*
*Am I speaking at a comforting pace and tone?*

---

Tone, pace, clarity, silence, soft tone, and emphasis all contribute, to the way you communicate. Consider how you express words and what factors might impinge on your ability to do this compassionately. Develop a calming soothing compassionate tone of voice. Think of the most compassionate sounding voice you know and name what it is about that voice that makes it so. Practice using it as often as you can.

## Non-verbal (Eye contact, touch, facial expression)

In addition to communicating through speech, we use our bodies to express ourselves to others. This is called non-verbal communication and is expressed through gestures, touch, appearance, eye contact, and facial expressions. It is also referred to as body language. As the saying goes, first impressions last. Projecting an image of professionalism can have a massive impact on clients and patients. This usually occurs unconsciously and is involuntary. It is estimated that between 55% and 95% of our communication is non-verbal. The way we do this sends a message to those around us. We might not even realise that we are doing it. Such as saying that we are okay when our body language gives the opposite message. It is important to understand the ways we express ourselves through our body language conveys compassion to the patient, and equally how they express themselves to us. Equally, looking at how your clients speak to you using their bodies can show how they are feeling.

---

**BOX 7.3  NON-VERBAL**

Ask yourself:

*Am I comfortable with eye contact?*
*Do my facial expressions/body match my words?*

---

Things to consider are open body language, facial expression, eye contact, touch, proximity, and gestures. Be aware that being close to someone can be comforting, but it can also make another feel uncomfortable. Know when to move forward and when to back off. Smiling is an excellent way to convey warmth and understanding, as is a concerned look when the client is speaking. Holdings someone's hand to express comfort or concern adds to this. Body language can be extra helpful when trying to convey compassion wearing a mask. What are the ways you can do this?

> *Think space, place, and face – body proximity, location, and facial expressions.*

Something you can try to develop your ability to understand what someone is saying without words is to watch a TV show, film with the volume off, and see if you can decipher the non-verbal messages being given by the speaker. You could even try this with people in public, from a suitable distance of course.

## Active Listening

Active listening is the way we respond to what is being said to us after hearing the full message. It includes verbally communicating an understanding of what has been said and asking questions. Effective use of open questions can make a massive difference in the dialogue between practitioner and patient, and as the name suggests open up opportunities for exploration and discovery. Answers to closed questions on the other hand can be yes or no. While they can be helpful when looking for straightforward answers, they limit what the practitioner can learn about their client or patient.

---

**BOX 7.4  ACTIVE LISTENING**

Ask yourself:

*Do I consider myself a good listener?*
*What is it about me that makes me a good listener?*

---

Being attentive, blocking out distractions, mindful focus, listen for meaning. Check in with yourself and ask what I am missing, and what are they saying. Try to remain calm when they are speaking and wait to respond to what they have said.

## Simple exercise - listening with compassion (adapted from Neff & Germer, 2018)

One of the hallmarks of compassionate communication is being present with the person's story. Our minds can easily be distracted especially if the client or patients story is distressing and creates overwhelming feelings in you. A helpful exercise for this is compassionate listening. The exercise has two parts, embodied listening and giving and receiving compassion. Try this out next time you are listening to a client or patients distressing story.

Embodied listening – in this step try to listen with your whole body. Let whatever you are feeling be present in that moment as well as seeing how they speak and listening to what they are saying. If you can, try to radiate compassion for them and yourself if you feel uncomfortable. Aim to hold it so that you can really listen to what the speaker is telling you.

Giving and receiving compassion – If you find that your attention has wandered, just bring your focus back to your breath, breathing compassion in for yourself and compassion out for the other person. This will help reconnect you to yourself and the speaker. This can also help you fight the urge to interrupt or offer a solution to their problem. Also, try not to put too much of your attention on your breathing but just enough to ground you in the moment without losing sight of the speaker's message.

## A compassionate communication checklist

**TABLE 7.1** Things to consider and practice when communicating to a patient or client

| Mouth (Speaking) | Yes | No |
| --- | --- | --- |
| Have you introduced yourself? Hello, my name is … | | |
| Have you told them the purpose of your conversation? | | |
| Have you checked to understand? | | |
| Did you interrupt them? | | |
| Are you aware of any language barriers?? | | |
| Is your tone right for the message? | | |
| **Ears (Listening)** | | |
| Have you listened to the full message? | | |
| Have you reduced distractions? | | |
| Is the room you are in suitable for communication? | | |

(*Continued*)

**TABLE 7.1** (Continued)

| Body (Non-verbal) | Yes | No |
|---|---|---|
| Does your body language match your words? | | |
| Can the person see you? | | |
| Is your body language open? | | |
| Are you making appropriate eye contact? | | |
| Does your facial expression match the message you are conveying? | | |
| Have you left enough personal space between you and the patient? | | |
| Are you expressing emotion and empathy through touch? | | |

## Summary

### Definition

Communication is defined as the expression of compassion through verbal and non-verbal interactions between self and patient, through tone of voice, body language/posture, eye contact, and effective listening. Using this strength to express and respond with compassion in ways that make the patient feels listened to.

### Key indicators

Verbal, Body language, Listening

### Psychology

We can communicate using all three psychologies. We can communicate using our body language, verbalise our emotions, think about what we are saying, and listen with compassion.

### Evidenced by

The display of compassionate verbal and non-verbal communication, supportive tone and actively listening to a patient's concerns no matter how small.

### Prevalence of this strength

Communication is another highly thought compassion strength. How you speak, listen, and convey understanding is key to compassion.

## Reflective questions

*What am I currently doing or can do to show this strength in myself (and others)?*
*In what ways does my communication demonstrate compassion?*
*How are my listening skills?*
*What tone do I use to convey compassionate understanding?*

## Combing strengths

**Communication** goes well with **empathy, Interpersonal skills, self-care, and connection**, in that it helps raise our awareness of needs, we can communicate to ourselves how we are feeling, empathise with that feeling, recognise and connect to what we need, and treat ourselves with compassion and care.

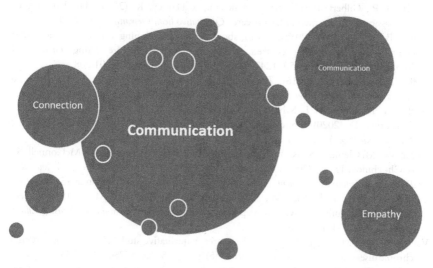

**FIGURE 7.1**  How communication combines with other compassion strengths

## Conclusion

In this chapter, we have explored the compassion strength of communication. Communication is one of the most important strengths. It is an effective method of expressing compassion, understanding of the patient's concerns, and suffering. Without it, we would not get extremely far in our attempts to help and support others. There are many ways in which we can communicate, and all must be used to fully achieve our goals of compassionate consideration of the other. As it is something you do daily, practice how you communicate with everyone you meet each day. Focus on your tone, body language, the words you use, and the way you listen. It might just make the difference.

What have you learned that you did not know before?

_____

_____

_____

_____

_____

## References

Bramley, L., & Matiti, M. (2014). How does it really feel to be in my shoes? Patients' experiences of compassion within nursing care and their perceptions of developing compassionate nurses. *Journal of Clinical Nursing, 23,* 2790–2799. 10.1111/jocn.12537

Coiera, E. (2006). Communication systems in healthcare. *The Clinical Biochemist. Reviews, 27*(2), 89–98.

Crawford, P., Gilbert, P., Gilbert, J., Gale, C., & Harvey, K. (2013). The language of compassion in acute mental health care. *Qualitative health research, 23*(6), 719–727.

Dewar, B., & Nolan, M. (2013). Caring about caring: Developing a model to implement compassionate relationship centred care in an older people care setting. *International Journal of Nursing Studies, 50,* 1247–1258. 10.1016/j.ijnurstu.2013.01.008

Neff, K., & Germer, C. (2018). *The Mindful Self-Compassion Workbook: A Proven Way to Accept Yourself, Build Inner Strength, and Thrive.* Guilford Publications.

Sinclair, S., Kondejewski, J., Schulte, F., Letourneau, N., Kuhn, S., Raffin-Bouchal, S., ... & Strother, D. (2020). Compassion in pediatric healthcare: a scoping review. *Journal of Pediatric Nursing, 51,* 57–66.

Sinclair, S., McClement, S., Raffin-Bouchal, S., Hack, T. F., Hagen, N. A., McConnell, S., & Chochinov, H. M. (2016). Compassion in health care: An empirical model. *Journal of Pain and Symptom Management, 51*(2), 193–203. 10.1016/j.jpainsymman.2015.10.009

Tehranineshat, B., Rakhshan, M., Torabizadeh, C., & Fararouei, M. (2018). Nurses', patients', and family caregivers' perceptions of compassionate nursing care. *Nursing Ethics.* 10.1177/0969733018777884

Van der Cingel, M. (2011). Compassion in care: A qualitative study of older people with a chronic disease and nurses. *Nursing Ethics, 18*(5), 672–685. 10.1177%2F0969733011403556

Way, D., & Tracy, S. J. (2012). Conceptualizing compassion as recognizing, relating and (re) acting: A qualitative study of compassionate communication at hospice. *Communication Monographs, 79,* 292–315. 10.1080/03637751.2012.697630

# 8

# COMPASSIONATE CHARACTER

## Introduction

These exercises are based on the development of compassionate character. Our character is important for how we present ourselves and behave with clients, patients, service users, their family and friends, and our colleagues. In this chapter you will learn:

1. What we mean by compassionate character
2. The opposites of compassionate character
3. Why we need compassionate character in healthcare
4. The obstacles to compassionate character
5. The types of compassionate character

## What is compassionate character?

Compassionate character refers to the behaviours and actions that make someone compassionate. It is related to virtues and how individuals conduct themselves doing for others in their work and community. Virtues are character traits that people use to do and be good. Things that take truly little thought to conclude that they are good. They come naturally to us, such as knowing that kindness and honesty are good things. Compassionate character is a significant predictor of compassionate behaviour (Durkin et al., 2022). Character is different from personality in that personality is more noticeable while character comes out in different and more specific situations. Character differs from personality in that your character is established through a set of moral beliefs and reveals itself in certain interactions and experiences, whereas

DOI: 10.4324/9781003276425-8

personality is more visible. Equally, character is more fluid and easier to change as opposed to personality which is rigid and fixed.

Our character tends to be shaped by beliefs and virtues and is more malleable than the personality traits we are born with. Character evolved to adapt our personality to certain situations so that we could survive and benefit from them. For example, a naturally shy person might change themselves and become more confident at public speaking for work or to gain the attention of a potential romantic partner. Character is associated with a person's moral, social, and religious attributes that contribute to their behaviour. As a compassion strength, character can be defined as the common characteristics that one displays when expressing compassion to self and others. However, it takes more than knowing what it means to be a good person. It requires action of compassion through the characteristics associated with being compassionate. It also takes daily practice to turn these characteristics and the others presented in the model, into habits and strengths.

## The opposite of compassionate character

The opposite of compassionate character is characteristics such as greed, anger, hostility, envy, meanness, selfishness, and coldness. They all can limit the compassion shown to another person and make us unhappy. They can lead us down paths that do not help when we are trying to address people's concerns or help with suffering. However, the golden mean of character applies here. For example, someone who is too honest becomes blunt and their harsh words can do more damage than good. In healthcare, this is key to how practitioners communicate. Being cold or judgmental can also hinder effective compassionate care and be seen as a weakness of compassion rather than a strength.

## Why do we need compassionate character?

Florence Nightingale once said that a good nurse was someone who had cultivated virtues and qualities of the character to make them compassionate (Bradshaw, 2011). While she was referring specifically to nurses, the same applies to all helping professions. The character of any healthcare practitioner and student is key to their delivery of effective compassionate care. Knowing what these characteristics are and how not only to identify but develop them is the purpose of this section of the book. You may already have and demonstrate these attributes, or you may want to learn more about them. Either way, this chapter will introduce and discuss the qualities that make someone compassionate and underpin the other strengths in this book. Compassionate character can be shown through kind actions, behaviours, and words, or a silent caring and respectful attitude. It can aid in understanding between practitioner and patient. The practitioner cannot truly support or help the client if their values and attitude toward others are not based on compassion. How can an indifferent, uncaring, and disrespectful practitioner achieve this? They may show highly skilled clinical abilities and knowledge but even though this is helpful and a form of compassion contingent on the situation, the patient still wants to feel cared for. They want to feel as though they are not just another patient but an individual with diverse needs, one's different to the last person you saw before them. They want to be listened to, understood, and treated with dignity, kindness, warmth, and honesty. People who express warmth are viewed as being friendly, kind, and helpful (Fiske et al., 2019). A person who is said to be soothing will be doing this with warmth. Patients feel understood when they are treated with warmth. It is considered the difference between the practitioner who knows what they are doing (competence), and knowing the patients (Howe et al., 2019).

## Obstacles to compassionate character

There are obstacles to compassionate character such as those listed below. These things vary in their degree and range of preventing practitioners from expressing their compassionate character, so they are presented as suggestions, not facts.

> *Feeling rushed*
> *Being self-orientated*
> *Being more clinical*
> *A neutral approach to care*
> *A coldness about the practitioner*
> *Neuroticism*
> *Hostility*

What other things get in your way?

_____
_____
_____
_____
_____

How motivated do you feel on a scale of 1 (not much), to 10 (very much) to use your compassionate characteristics, such as courage and kindness with self and others.

Self: _____

Others: _____

## The evidence for character and compassion

Your beliefs about care and compassion, and the people who are deserving of it can shape the character and behaviours you present when with clients or patients. This is motivated by internal desires, beliefs, and attitudes that shape the behaviour towards being good and doing good for others. We associate character and virtues with morality and altruism, with our need to help others being as equally bene-ficial for them as they are rewarding for us. To be truly compassionate one must own the mental state and motivations that drive them toward acts of compassion. Courage for instance motivates us to move toward our own and the suffering of others, rather than away from it. Compassionate character is linked with good character and doing the right thing because it is morally so. For healthcare practitioners to be considered compassionate they must have, develop, and show the qualities of a compassionate person.

Bradshaw (2011) states that "Compassion is grounded in the "quality of an individual's character". It can be demonstrated through acts of warmth (Bray et al., 2014), genuineness, and kindness (Kneafsey et al., 2015). Honesty, trust, value, respect, sympathy, openness, kindness, genuineness, authenticity, acceptance, and loving concern are important qualities for a compassionate practitioner to have (Sinclair et al., 2016b). In a study involving Dutch nurses, compassion was pre-dicated on a helping attitude (Van der Cingel, 2011).

Character is concerned with the virtues and behaviours people show with others. Healthcare practitioners see how a caring attitude or behaviour is key for patients at the time of intense suffering (Su et al., 2020). Similarly, positive psychology seeks to help individuals find their own unique set of character strengths and provide the conditions that cultivate their growth (Linkins et al., 2015). An ardent desire to care for others, and being cooperative, dependable, and tolerant are just some of the personal qualities that drive individuals to become helpers (Eley et al., 2010). Being truthful, and other personal characteristics of care, flexibility, and respect for self and others, contribute to the idea of a "good nurse" who does "the right thing" (Smith & Godfrey, 2002), and acts compassionately (Begley, 2010). Being kind for instance is associated with positive well-being (Hui et al., 2020). Indeed, nurses report that their compassionate behaviour is determined by their values and characteristics (Nijboer & Van der Cingel, 2018). The moral aspect of this combines attentiveness, and vulnerability with the courage to act on one's principles when facing the un-predictable. In doing so, practitioners overcome the barriers to providing compas-sionate care (Lindh et al., 2009). Dignity and respect are two of the main character traits promoted in staff who work in the NHS.

## Types of compassionate character

Compassionate character can be categorised into two distinct types. One concerns the actual behaviours and virtuous actions that practitioners use to show com-passion to others. The other is about virtuous expression and metaphysical aspects of the person that we do not see but know by their being that they are com-passionate. We can look at compassionate character as both including virtuous actions and behaviours, and virtuous being and expression. Being clear on these characteristics of compassion can help us understand what it is that they look like and thus what we can do to develop and show it in practice.

## Virtuous action

This type of compassionate character is concerned with the actual acts of compassion and how practitioners express their inner character. It is associated with kindness, being helpful, and friendly, having a soothing nature, using humour appropriately, and being generous with others. For example, kindness is defined as doing good for others, helping, and taking care of them. It is associated with nurturing, generosity, care, altruism, and being nice (Peterson & Seligman, 2004).

---

**BOX 8.1  VIRTUOUS ACTION**

Things to ask yourself:

*How helpful am I to patients?*
*In what ways am I kind to others?*
*How do I use my virtuous action with clients and patients?*

---

## Courage

Courage is a key characteristic of a compassionate person. It gives us the strength to engage with another's pain as well as our own. When showing courage, we allow ourselves to be open and vulnerable to suffering so that we can attend to it with our other compassionate qualities.

## Kindness

Kindness can help alleviate the discomfort you feel when witnessing another person's situation. Show kindness to your clients/patients as well as your colleagues. Be generous with others, with your time, and how you support people. You may have heard of random acts of kindness.

## Simple exercise

Think about what you can do today (and each day) for others with a simple random act of kindness in your practice. They can be big or small and to whoever you wish. Try at least five acts of kindness a day. This will make people feel good and increase your well-being too.

1. _____
2. _____
3. _____
4. _____
5. _____

## Care

A caring person is someone who does what is necessary to support the health and wellbeing of another person. Care can be expressed through actions and words and goes hand in hand with other compassion strengths such as communication and engagement. Think of ways you can bring your strengths together when caring for others.

## Encouraging

Use encouraging words to create optimism and hope. Be realistic with what you are encouraging others to do but aim to be positive in your outlook. This can help create a positive self-fulfilling prophecy where the others believe in you and themselves.

## Friendly

Although you do not have to become friends with patients and clients you can still be friendly. Show interest in them and treat them as someone you accept and respect just because they are human. Be as friendly as possible. Ask questions, using a soothing tone.

## Helpful

Help others whenever you can, whether that is your clients' patients, their families, or colleagues. Being helpful can take on various forms. We will look at how you can go over and beyond in the chapter on engagement.

## Adaptable

Being adaptable is linked to resilience and a skill that can be developed. There will be times when you are expected to do extra work or something that is outside of your comfort zone. Although it might feel uncomfortable at first, your ability to adapt to different situations will help you grow the strength needed to take this on.

## Reliable

Being reliable and keeping any promises you make can benefit your clients as well as your colleagues. If people know that you will deliver on what you say you will then they will be more likely to turn to you in times of need.

## Honesty

Honesty is about being honest and authentic both with others and with yourself. Congruence with who you are and how you act is especially important. Be honest about what you can or cannot do. Know your limits. Reassure your client/patient about any concerns they may have but be realistic. Honesty when delivered gently is perceived as kind and compassionate, especially when telling someone bad news such as they have cancer (Berry et al., 2017).

## Virtuous expression

This type of character is associated with the parts of being that cannot be seen directly but are compassionate, such as showing warmth, being honest, authentic, respectful, and thoughtful. It is about tolerance and being trusting of others. Someone hopeful. Compassion is driven by hope in that the practitioner wants their client or patient to not be suffering and to overcome their misfortune and distress.

---

**BOX 8.2  VIRTUOUS EXPRESSION**

Things to ask yourself:

*How tolerant am I of others?*
*In what ways do I express warmth?*
*How do I inspire hope in others?*

---

## Warmth

Warmth is a part of compassionate character that is linked to connection and empathy. By communicating warmth, the client knows that they will be treated with dignity and respect. Warmth is a pro-social characteristic. We are often judged by our character and warmth is no exception. It is associated with patient satisfaction, positive emotions, and behaviours.

## Respect

Be respectful to patients, their families, and your colleagues. By doing so you show that you value them as a person and that they matter to you regardless of their flaws. This helps build trust between patient and practitioner.

## Humility

Be humble. Although you might know all there is to know about your practice, clinical skills, or conditions, you do not know everything about the patient and their condition. This way you grow through the continuous stream of learning and upskilling. This is linked to a growth mindset.

## Hope

How does hope fit into compassion? Hope can be shown through expressing positive outcomes and hope for the present situation and the future. Think about how you do or can show hope for others.

## Humour

The use of appropriate humour and silliness has been shown to patient ease stress and worry. Laughter releases feel-good hormones which are linked to faster improvements in health and to the acceptance of each situation one finds themselves in. A good example of this is Patch Adams. Look into his story, see his talks on YouTube, or watch the film to get a sense of his philosophy behind humour as an antidote to suffering and the human connection between patient and practitioner.

## Gratitude

Express gratitude towards others, especially patients or clients who share sensitive information with you. Be thankful for the blessing you have been given and the work that you do. Express this in ways that work for you. A journal, in your mind or outwardly to others. Give thanks openly to those you are grateful for and what they bring into your life.

## Being open

This can be expressed through your body language and verbal communication. Being open helps the other person know more about you and is a way to establish boundaries for yourself. This not only protects you from burnout but creates a clear idea of what you will and will not do or can do.

## Understanding

Having an understanding character not only makes you more approachable but protects you from being judgemental. Thinking beyond what the person presents with to someone who is suffering or has suffered is key to being compassionate.

## Accepting

Accepting others is linked to tolerance and other strengths such as empathy. By seeing things from the other person's perspective irrespective of what has happened to them or what they have done, you can become more accepting of them as a human being.

## Authentic

Linked to congruence, being authentic means being your true self with others. This might leave you open and vulnerable, but it will make you more self-aware and focused on being who you are. When our authentic self is present, we inadvertently allow others to show their true selves. Being authentic is linked to other aspects of compassionate character such as reliability.

## Simple exercise – identifying your compassionate character

What are your top 5 compassionate characteristics?

1. _____
2. _____
3. _____
4. _____
5. _____

## Summary

### Definition

Character is associated with a person's moral, social, and religious attributes that contribute to their behaviour. As a compassion strength, character can be defined as the common characteristics that one displays when expressing compassion to self and others.

### Key indicators

The key indicators of these strengths are Kindness, Care, Acceptance, Honesty, Humour, Warmth, Respect, Trust, Authentic, and Loving concern.

### Psychology

This strength covers all three aspects of behaviour, emotion, and cognitive. For example, care and kindness can be expressed through behaviours, warmth with emotional expression, and respect through our thoughts.

### Evidenced by

The display of personal positive virtues and character with patient (client/service user) family, friends, colleagues, and towards self.

### Prevalence of that strength

Students, practitioners, educators, and service users view character as one of the top compassion strengths for practitioners to demonstrate to their patients. For, how one presents themselves can be just as if not more important for patients than the care they receive.

### Reflective questions

Think about this strength and the parts of your character you demonstrate in your practice. Are they different outside of work?

*What am I currently doing or can do to demonstrate this strength in myself and others? What are my negative traits and characteristics that I would like to avoid?*

### Combing strengths

Character is strengthened when it is combined with all other strengths. Character sits central to other aspects of compassion as it is the driving force behind our behaviour and actions. You can bring together both aspects of your compassionate character in various settings.

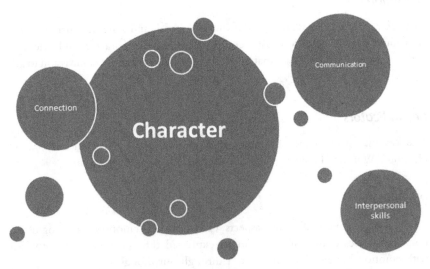

**FIGURE 8.1** How character combines with other compassion strengths

## Conclusion

In this chapter we have explored what character is, what it is not, why it is important, and the different kinds of compassionate character. Character is another central aspect of compassion strengths, as it is about you and the parts of your being that define who you are. The wonderful thing about character is that we can change and mould ourselves into something new. It is through this respect to let our compassionate side shine through.

What have you learned that you did not know before?

_____

_____

_____

_____

_____

# References

Begley, A. M. (2010). On being a good nurse: reflections on the past and preparing for the future. *International Journal of Nursing Practice, 16*(6), 525–532. 10.1111/j.1440-172X.2010. 01878.x

Berry, L. L., Danaher, T. S., Chapman, R. A., & Awdish, R. L. (2017). Role of kindness in cancer care. *Journal of Oncology Practice, 13*(11), 744–750.

Bradshaw, A. (2011). Compassion: what history teaches us. *Nursing Times, 107*(19–20), 12–14.

Bray, L., O'Brien, M. R., Kirton, J., Zubairu, K., & Christiansen, A. (2014). The role of professional education in developing compassionate practitioners: A mixed methods study exploring the perceptions of health professionals and pre-registration students. *Nurse Education Today, 34*, 480–486. 10.1016/j.nedt.2013.06.017

Durkin, M., Gurbutt, R., & Carson, J. (2022). Effectiveness of an online short compassion strengths course on nursing students compassion: A mixed methods non-randomised pilot study. *Nurse Education Today, 111*, 105315.

Eley, R., Eley, D., & Rogers-Clark, C. (2010). Reasons for entering and leaving nursing: an Australian regional study. *Australian Journal of Advanced Nursing, 28*(1), 6–13.

Fiske, S. T., Cuddy, A. J., Peter, G., & Xu, J. (2019). "A model of (often mixed) stereotype content: Competence and warmth respectively follow from perceived status and competition": Correction to Fiske et al. (2002). *Journal of Personality and Social Psychology.* 10.1037/pspa0000163

Howe, L. C., Leibowitz, K. A., & Crum, A. J. (2019). When your doctor "Gets It" and "Gets You": The critical role of competence and warmth in the patient–provider interaction. *Frontiers in psychiatry, 475.*

Hui, B. P., Ng, J. C., Berzaghi, E., Cunningham-Amos, L. A., & Kogan, A. (2020). Rewards of kindness? A meta-analysis of the link between prosociality and well-being. *Psychological Bulletin, 146*(12), 1084.

Kneafsey, R., Brown, S., Sein, K., Chamley, C., & Parsons, J. (2015). A qualitative study of key stakeholders' perspectives on compassion in healthcare and the development of a framework for compassionate interpersonal relations. *Journal of Clinical Nursing, 25*, 70–79. 10.1111/jocn.12964

Lindh, I. B., Severinsson, E., & Berg, A. (2009). Nurses' moral strength: A hermeneutic inquiry in nursing practice. *Journal of Advanced Nursing, 65*(9), 1882–1890. 10.1111/j.13 65-2648.2009.05047.x

Linkins, M., Niemiec, R. M., Gillham, J., & Mayerson, D. (2015). Through the lens of strength: A framework for educating the heart. *The Journal of Positive Psychology, 10*(1), 64–68. 10.1080/17439760.2014.888581

Nijboer, A. A., & Van der Cingel, M. C. J. M. (2018). Compassion: Use it or lose it? A study into the perceptions of novice nurses on compassion: A qualitative approach. *Nurse Education Today*, *72*, 84–89.

Peterson, C., & Seligman, M. E. (2004). *Character strengths and virtues: A handbook and classification* (Vol. 1). Oxford University Press.

Sinclair, S., McClement, S., Raffin-Bouchal, S., Hack, T. F., Hagen, N. A., McConnell, S., & Chochinov, H. M. (2016b). Compassion in health care: An empirical model. *Journal of Pain and Symptom Management*, *51*(2), 193–203. 10.1016/j.jpainsymman.2015.10.009

Smith, K. V., & Godfrey, N. S. (2002). Being a good nurse and doing the right thing: a qualitative study. *Nursing Ethics*, *9*(3), 301–312. 10.1191/0969733002ne512oa

Su, J. J., Masika, G. M., Paguio, J. T., & Redding, S. R. (2020). Defining compassionate nursing care. *Nursing ethics*, *27*(2), 480–493. 10.1177%2F0969733019851546

Van der Cingel, M. (2011). Compassion in care: A qualitative study of older people with a chronic disease and nurses. *Nursing Ethics*, *18*(5), 672–685. 10.1177%2F0969733011403556

# 9

# CONNECTION

## Introduction

Human connection is fundamental to our development and wellbeing. We need other people to thrive and stay alive. Without others, we can become isolated and closed off to the world, opportunities, and experiences that might help us grow. This chapter will cover some of the numerous ways connection can be achieved by practitioners and the different types of connections that you can use to connect with your patients.

In this chapter you will learn:

1. What we mean by connection
2. The opposites of connection
3. Why we need connection in healthcare
4. The obstacles to this compassion strengths
5. The types of connection

## What is connection?

Human connection is a deep bond developed between two people in which one or both feel heard, understood, valued, and seen. It helps foster trust as well as the positive energy that comes from feeling connected to someone. Maslow (1962) considered connection as being next level to food, water, shelter, and safety. Having close relationships and connecting to other human beings is better for our well-being and survival than physical activity, avoiding smoking or air pollution (Uchino, 2006). This makes sense from an evolutionary perspective as our ancestors would have received help from close contact with others to aid in their survival. Working together to provide shelter, food, comfort, and safety from stress

DOI: 10.4324/9781003276425-9

or brief life-threatening events meant that we survived and lived to grow, raise children, develop, and see another day. Having strong connections at work with both patients and colleagues can help reduce burnout, develop communication and learning and overall provide more efficient care. It taps into our shared humanity and brings us closer together.

## The opposite of connection

The opposite of connection is loneliness, isolation, and disconnection. These can make someone feel unfulfilled both mentally, physically, and spiritually. Being alone can increase the release of the stress hormone cortisol, with chronic stress associated with a higher risk of heart disease and stroke. Not being seen, known, or heard can make people closed off and uncared for. Feeling that you are disconnected from others, especially during times of great need, can be a horrible experience.

## Why we need connection in healthcare

Rather than just another body, patients had a past, future, stories, hopes, and dreams. They need to feel that they are more than an illness or condition and be greeted and spoken to as fellow human beings. For example, historically, mental health issues have been considered an illness of the mind and brain. Because of this view, patients and service users have been treated as though there is something up with them without considering their background. However, more recently, psychologists have questioned this line of thinking and instead proposed that practitioners explore the experiences which have led to this and rather than thinking what is up with this person, ask them "what happened to you?" (Johnstone & Boyle, 2018). This can help you connect to the person on a personal level and understand how their experiences have shaped their lives. While it is not always practical or necessary to gain insight into somebody's back story, at the fundamental level, there is more benefit than harm in asking the patient questions to get to know them a little. Connection from the patient's perspective helps them be known in a meaningful way (Thorne et al., 2005). It is linked to other compassion strengths such as communication and empathy and is key to shaping the patient's experience of care. Human connection helps patients be seen as other human beings, and the person beneath the disease or condition. It acknowledges that there is more to care than clinal competence and that through compassion patients and practitioners can be vulnerable. People are more than just their problems or suffering. Connection honours the humanness in each of us and empowers patients during their care.

## Obstacles to this strength

*Distance due to online technology*
*Language and cultural barriers*

*Being unfocused*
*Physical barriers*
*Inability to form connections*
*No common ground*
*They may have had a bad experience with others in a similar role*

What other things get in your way?

_____

_____

_____

_____

_____

How motivated do you feel on a scale of 1 (not much), to 10 (very much) to create a compassionate connection with self and others?

Self: _____

Others: _____

## The evidenced based benefits of connection and compassion

Connection is another key compassion strength that enhances the practitioner-patient dynamic. The ability to connect to patients is considered central to compassionate care (Newham et al., 2017), and considered one of the many privileges of working in the helping professions. It is through the connection that nursing students learn about the significance of humanised compassionate care and the fundamental aspects that make it possible (Scammell, 2016). A feature of this is a spiritual dimension of nursing care, which enables nurses to connect with patients in a profound manner (Golberg, 1998). Formulating human connections, helps patients feel validated, and the nurse to be more comfortable with another's experience. Enabling patients to "become known" as an individual with their unique problems, has a profound healing effect between practitioner and patient (Thorne et al., 2005). When taught about connection, nursing students learn how to honour the quality of life and gain respect for patients in their care, in addition to becoming more self-aware and complicit in their care (De Natale & Klevay, 2013). Putting the patient's needs first is viewed as a compassion quality (Sinclair, 2016a). According to both patients and practitioners, having a presence or being there is one of the most important qualities of a compassionate nurse (Van der Cingel, 2011). It is also a motivating factor for physicians to both demonstrate compassion and protect themselves from burnout (Branch et al., 2017).

Meaningful connection features as a core element of compassion for midwives that helps them recognise each woman's needs and support them during childbirth. How the midwife cares for the mother relies on personal and cultural awareness of her and her family. This requires compassionate connection as well as competency. This along with characteristics such as respect, trust, interpersonal skills, and empathy, enables a compassionate caring collaboration between the midwife and the woman in labour (Krausé et al., 2020).

Connection is an effective method of getting to know patients at a deeper level in order to gain a better understanding of their needs. Clients, patients, and service users see connection as a significant and highly sought-after characteristic of a compassionate practitioner. Connecting with patients using humour, sharing personal stories, and warmth is crucial for seeing them as a person rather than just an illness (Dewar & Nolan, 2013; Kret, 2011; Peters, 2006). By getting to know them on a deeper level, connection becomes the vehicle that helps practitioners understand suffering, and care for patients in ways they want to be cared for. Taking time, empathising, and using interpersonal communication skills with patients are methods that when combined increase the opportunity for connections to evolve. This is reminiscent of a humanistic approach to care. Learning how to become proficient in this is considered necessary for demonstrating compassion.

Nurturing a natural humanistic connection toward patients is considered compassionate (Peters, 2006). Badger and Royse (2012) found that patients recalled feeling like a person when a nurse said good morning to them. Bramley and Matiti (2014) found that getting to know the patient helped nurses understand each patient's individual needs. Patients report feeling genuinely cared for when staff members connected with them or gave them their full attention (Kneafsey et al., 2015). This attentiveness coupled with respecting their dignity and privacy was also noted by Bray et al. (2014). The value of this was highlighted by Dewar and Nolan (2013) as establishing a shared understanding with the patient, identifying their needs, guided by curiosity, fosters a humble approach to patient care. Indeed, if they cannot understand the emotional and psychological states of their patients, nurses feel that they cannot be compassionate (Tehranineshat et al., 2018). Being attentive was reported by Kret (2011) as the second highest identified theme for qualities of a compassionate nurse.

Being aware of the patient's context such as experiencing a lack of independence, financial constraints, or emotional or family issues, is a way of demonstrating compassion (Sinclair et al., 2016a). Involvement in the patient's suffering helps create bonds between practitioner and patient (Van der Cingel (2011). Showing how these strengths link to the strength of competence, Lee and Seomun (2016) reported that professional knowledge helped give the nurse more insight into a patient's condition and heightened their awareness of suffering. Sinclair (2016) and Way and Tracy (2012) noted that compassion also meant addressing the patient's suffering and improve well-being which could be achieved by getting to know the patient through empathy and communication. A key facilitator of connection is cultural competence. Understanding the person's cultural and ethnic background can help provide care in a way that is meaningful to that person and respects their culture and beliefs.

## Types of connection

We can break connection down into two key types. One is knowing the patient and the other is awareness of needs and suffering. They are linked to presence and the therapeutic relationship, which form the foundation of being known.

## Knowing the patient

Knowing the patient is about connecting to the patient, and who they are. It is about the present and how the practitioner uses their other compassion strengths such as communication and engagement to relate and get to know the person within the patient, what makes them tick, and what they are about. It takes purposive intent on the practitioner's behalf to connect with the patient and achieve results that are beneficial for both. Take time before you meet a client or patient, to get to know a bit about their background. Use this to prepare, connect and learn more about them. Consider their cultural background, their beliefs about suffering, being sick, and what care means to them.

---

**BOX 9.1   KNOWING THE PATIENT**

Things to ask yourself:

*How well do I know my patient/client?*
*How connected am I to the whole person?*
*How can I contribute to the patient's journey?*

---

Simply acknowledging the person and letting them know that you see them, you know who they are, that they matter, and you care about them are ways to demonstrate human connection. Equally, ask about them, where they are from, do they have family, kids, husbands, wives, and parents. See small talk to get to know them on a personal level. What do they do for work? If they are retired, what did they do? Do they study? If they are too young to have a job, how is school? Or if they are unemployed, ask what they would like to do. Remember, each person is different.

While their condition might be similar, the path that led them to you will surely not. They have unique lives that are full of memories of experiences that have been felt by them in ways that are fundamentally different from everyone else. Wanting to learn about your patient will help make them feel they meant something to you. Try at that moment, to make them feel that they are your only patient. Get to know their name. Something as simple as this can forge that connection. Remembering their name and information associated with their case will strengthen the human connection even more. Letting them refer to you by your first name rather than a title can add to this in ways that bring both practitioner and patient to an equal level.

This type of connection relates to the compassionate character of curiosity. Share something about yourself that can help break down any barriers that might exist between you. However, bear in mind the context of disclosure and the amount of information you share. Crying with them during challenging times and being elated when good news comes, are also ways to forge a human connection with the people you treat. Overall use your unique humanness to develop your strengths of compassionate connection.

Connecting to the whole person involves seeing the whole person as not just the condition or illness, but as someone with their values, beliefs, culture, and emotional, spiritual, physical, and psychological needs. Their individual preferences and care needs. People need to feel validated by their experiences and suffering. There it is important to do this for clients/patients on more than one level of connection. For example, their emotional state of mind will matter to them more than their physical state of being. Here, compassionate communication can help forge a connection when providing information about the person that might be uncomfortable for them to hear in the right way. Make it personal for them, taking into consideration their situation, background and condition or illness, and with what they are struggling.

Find ways to connect to each part of their humanness. For example, you do not have to share the same beliefs but acknowledge that this means something to them. This can help create a strong bond between you and make them feel valued and validated. In certain cases, you will also have to connect to the patient's fears. They may be going through the worse experience of their life and will need to be treated with empathy, sympathy, and understanding. Being with them in more than a physical presence in their time of need can be powerful. This is about connecting to the patient's story. Being positive and using encouraging words can support this process. Praising them for their achievements, what steps they have made already, and their successes can be powerful forms of connection. Use this connection to help you become more aware of the patient's suffering and understand what their needs are and how you can support them.

Ask questions that are related to practice, such as "what brings you here today"? But also, ask about someone's tattoo, their favourite sports team, what brings them joy, and what makes them happy. Perspective attainment rather than taking. Using humour can be good to connect but must be done with thought and consideration of the other person. Showing genuine interest in their background is a way to connect compassionately. This allows for the increased awareness of their needs and how to respond to these unique requirements.

## Awareness of needs/suffering

To be compassionate it is important to first know what the other person is suffering from and what their needs are in any given situation. To do this one must focus on the patient, give them their full attention, and use other compassion strengths such as empathy, and active listening to connect and understand them fully. You want to understand their level of suffering, what might be causing it and how you can help them through it. We all suffer from something at certain times in our life. Having this common humanity brings us closer to that realisation and each other.

---

## BOX 9.2  AWARENESS OF NEEDS/SUFFERING

Things to ask yourself:

*What is this person suffering from?*
*What are their needs and what can I do to help them?*

---

Listen to the patient or client, and their families intently using empathy to connect to their pain. Use your strengths of compassionate communication to address and understand what they want and need from you. Noticing what they are telling you either explicitly or implicitly can create a connection and make them feel heard and understood. Talking through concerns and if there is a problem, figuring out how to solve it with them is an enormously powerful way to connect with them. Remove all distractions that can get in the way. This could be technology such as a phone or other electronic device, or form of physical distraction for example a chair. It is important to look at them and not at a screen when communicating with patients. Focusing on the patient helps foster a connection that aims to understand the person and their needs. Being mindful of them and your thoughts, feelings, and behaviours in that moment can aid with the connection. Listen to their story to learn and understand.

The practice of mindfulness can help people bring their attention to the present moment, focusing on the client, and the task at hand. It can help to take a moment before every interaction and pause to clear your mind and prepare for your next appointment. Washing your hands, a brief walk, getting a drink, or three deep breaths are small but effective ways to anchor yourself and prepare you for connecting to the next person, especially when time is against you. Understanding what matters most to a patient and their needs, is fundamental to person-centred care and the connection between practitioner and patient.

## Simple exercises – compassionate connections

A simple exercise you can do to help you develop your compassionate connections influenced by the work of Barbara Fredrickson, is to think about the micromoments of compassionate connection each day. At the end of each day, reflect on how "close", "in-tune" and compassionate you were with other people. Shifting your attention to each compassionate moment can lead to greater change and connection overtime. To do this, review your day, and pick out each of the compassionate connections you had and rate them for how in tune you were, how close you were, and how compassionate you were. Doing this on a daily basis can help you monitor and see changes in your compassionate connections. You will be able to notice when change occurred and what might have affected it.

## Summary

### Definition

A humanistic connection to the person behind the patient, client, or service user helps foster a deeply personal experience.

### Key indicators

Connecting to and knowing the patient, Awareness of needs/suffering

### Psychology

Because we can connect to others through the things we do, the emotions we share with them, and the shared thoughts we use all three psychologies.

### Evidenced by

Making the effort to know more about patients holistically as an individual with unique needs and experiences of ill health, and life.

### Prevalence of this strength

Seeing the patient as a person with a history present and future rather than someone with an issue that needs addressing is high up on the list of effective ways to show compassion.

### Reflective questions

*What am I currently doing or can do to demonstrate this strength in myself (and others)?*
*How do I connect to others?*
*What level of connection do I share with my patients, clients, service users, their families and
	friends, and my colleagues?*

### Combing strengths

To strengthen your connection, combine it with engagement, communication, and empathy to explore your client and forge a strong link between the two of you.

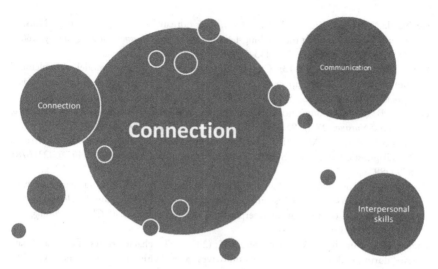

**FIGURE 9.1** How connection combines with other compassion strengths

## Conclusion

In this chapter, we have looked at connection as a compassion strength and how it is used to demonstrate compassion and a deeper level of understanding toward your patients and clients. Connection is particularly good at making the people you care for feel special, heard, and treated like human beings. It has benefits for you too so aim to connect often and reap the benefits of this compassion strength.

What have you learned that you did not know before?

_____

_____

_____

_____

_____

## References

Badger, K., & Royse, D. (2012). Describing compassionate care: the burn survivor's perspective. *Journal of Burn Care & Research, 33*, 772–780. 10.1097/BCR.0b013e318254d30b

Bramley, L., & Matiti, M. (2014). How does it really feel to be in my shoes? Patients' experiences of compassion within nursing care and their perceptions of developing compassionate nurses. *Journal of Clinical Nursing, 23*, 2790–2799. 10.1111/jocn.12537

Branch Jr, W. T., Weil, A. B., Gilligan, M. C., Litzelman, D. K., Hafler, J. P., Plews-Ogan, M., ..., & Frankel, R. M. (2017). How physicians draw satisfaction and overcome barriers in their practices: "It sustains me". *Patient Education and Counseling, 100*(12), 2320–2330.

Bray, L., O'Brien, M. R., Kirton, J., Zubairu, K., & Christiansen, A. (2014). The role of professional education in developing compassionate practitioners: A mixed methods study exploring the perceptions of health professionals and pre-registration students. *Nurse Education Today, 34*, 480–486. 10.1016/j.nedt.2013.06.017

De Natale, M. L., & Klevay, A. M. (2013). The human becoming connection: Nursing students find meaning in the teaching-learning processes. *Nursing Science Quarterly, 26*(2), 125–129. 10.1177%2F0894318413477148

Dewar, B., & Nolan, M. (2013). Caring about caring: Developing a model to implement compassionate relationship centred care in an older people care setting. *International Journal of Nursing Studies, 50*, 1247–1258. 10.1016/j.ijnurstu.2013.01.008

Golberg, B. (1998). Connection: an exploration of spirituality in nursing care. *Journal of Advanced Nursing, 27*(4), 836–842. 10.1046/j.1365-2648.1998.00596.x

Johnstone, L., & Boyle, M. (2018). The Power Threat Meaning Framework: An Alternative Nondiagnostic Conceptual System. *Journal of Humanistic Psychology*. 10.1177/0022167818793289

Kneafsey, R., Brown, S., Sein, K., Chamley, C., & Parsons, J. (2015). A qualitative study of key stakeholders' perspectives on compassion in healthcare and the development of a framework for compassionate interpersonal relations. *Journal of Clinical Nursing, 25*, 70–79. 10.1111/jocn.12964

Krausé, S. S., Minnie, C. S., & Coetzee, S. K. (2020). The characteristics of compassionate care during childbirth according to midwives: a qualitative descriptive inquiry. *BMC Pregnancy and Childbirth, 20*(1), 1–10.

Kret, D. D. (2011). The qualities of a compassionate nurse according to the perceptions of medical-surgical patients. *Medsurg Nursing, 20*(1), 29–36. Retrieved from https://search.proquest.com/docview/851871755?accountid=9653

Lee, Y., & Seomun, G. (2016). Compassion competence in nurses. *Advances in Nursing Science, 39*(2), E54–E66.

Maslow, A. H. (1962). *Toward a psychology of being*. Princeton: D. Van Nostrand Company

Newham, R., Terry, L., Atherley, S., Hahessy, S., Babenko-Mould, Y., Evans, M., …, & Cedar, S. (2017). A moral profession: Nurse educators' selected narratives of care and compassion. *Nursing Ethics*. 10.1177/0969733016687163

Peters, M. A. (2006). Compassion: An Investigation into the Experience of Nursing Faculty. *International Journal for Human Caring, 10*, 38–46.

Scammell, J. (2016). Compassionate Care. In Barker, S (Eds), *Psychology for Nursing and Healthcare Professionals: Developing Compassionate Care* (pp 67–94.). London: Sage.

Sinclair, S., Norris, J. M., McConnell, S. J., Chochinov, H. M., Hack, T. F., Hagen, N. A., …, & Bouchal, S. R. (2016). Compassion: a scoping review of the healthcare literature. *BMC Palliative Care, 15*, 193–203. 10.1186/s12904-016-0080-0

Tehranineshat, B., Rakhshan, M., Torabizadeh, C., & Fararouei, M. (2018). Nurses', patients', and family caregivers' perceptions of compassionate nursing care. *Nursing Ethics*. 10.1177/0969733018777884

Thorne, S. E., Kuo, M., Armstrong, E. A., McPherson, G., Harris, S. R., & Hislop, T. G. (2005). 'Being known': patients' perspectives of the dynamics of human connection in cancer care. Psycho-Oncology: Journal of the Psychological. *Social and Behavioral Dimensions of Cancer, 14*(10), 887–898. 10.1002/pon.945

Uchino, B. N. (2006). Social Support and Health: A Review of Physiological Processes Potentially Underlying Links to Disease Outcomes. *J Behav Med, 29*, 377–387. 10.1007/s10865-006-9056-5

Van der Cingel, M. (2011). Compassion in care: A qualitative study of older people with a chronic disease and nurses. *Nursing Ethics, 18*(5), 672–685. 10.1177%2F0969733011403556

Way, Deborah, & Tracy, Sarah J. (2012). Conceptualizing Compassion as Recognizing, Relating and (Re)acting: A Qualitative Study of Compassionate Communication at Hospice. Communication Monographs, 79, 292–315 10.1080/03637751.2012.697630

# 10

# ENGAGEMENT

## Introduction

These exercises are based on the development of compassionate engagement. Engagement refers to the way you can engage with the patient and exceed your regular work to support them. In this chapter you will learn:

1. What we mean by engagement
2. The opposites of engagement
3. Why we need engagement
4. The obstacles to engagement
5. The types of engagement

## What do we mean by engagement?

At its core, engagement means to be engaged in something or someone. While we might be more familiar with the term client engagement, which refers to the process of forming deep connections through interaction, participation, and decisions making, compassionate engagement relates to the things the practitioner does to show compassion and connect to their client or patient. Engagement is associated with the small acts of kindness, the little things that make the biggest difference to people, and going above and beyond your regular duties. Going out of your way to do something for someone can be rewarding for both the giver and receiver. We often hear people say, "enjoy the little things." This phrase is used so much that we can forget the true meaning behind it. In healthcare, "doing the little things" helps not only the client but you to feel better. It is linked to patient and practitioner satisfaction. We can appreciate the small things that happen to us, such as hearing good news, or that someone has achieved something. When someone goes

DOI: 10.4324/9781003276425-10

out of their way to do something for us, we feel good and appreciated. This strength is strongly associated with connection. These small but effective acts of compassion that go beyond the regular call of duty are considered central to improving patient wellbeing, and the characteristics of a compassionate practitioner. Like rapport building, empathy, communication, and connection can be used to get to know the patient and do something above and beyond regular care. We might go that extra mile for someone we know or a stranger. Regardless of who they are, this helps form a human connection and reminder of the good in people.

## The opposite of compassionate engagement

The opposite of compassionate engagement is disengagement or detachment from the patient. Not wanting to do more than is needed or go out of one's way for the other person. Doing little to connect with them. Being present but not motivated to support them further. Being disengaged from them as a person prevents connection and understanding. When we do not go out of our way for others, we show disinterest in them and can seem cold and indifferent to their needs.

## Why do we need engagement in healthcare?

Random acts of kindness which are closely related to engagement bring about the good in us. Doing trivial things for people can have a massive impact on them and you. The focus should be on more than the grandiose things. Simple acts can leave a long-lasting memory of kindness and compassion on the person receiving your goodwill. In this model, engagement refers to active participation in patient care by going the extra mile or providing the little things that matter most. It is described as the practitioner, always being available, friendly, warm, and cheerful, gentle and nothing being too much trouble for them (Kralik et al., 1997). Engagement can have a powerful impact on the effectiveness and empowerment of nurses (Spence Laschinger et al., 2009). Indeed, going the extra mile helps to improve the systems of care and improve patient outcomes (Raper, 2014). Engagement also relies on the subjective response of the practitioner and is associated with the emotional labour attached to caring (Henderson, 2001), which can either motivate or demotivate the individual to act (Keyko et al., 2016). More importantly, despite all the excellent work, competency, and skills practitioners use to provide care, patients and clients often remember the little things that made a difference to them and made them feel cared for and valued.

## Obstacles to this strength

*Not having enough time*
*Thinking that compassion requires grand acts*
*Being too busy*
*Not being focused on the other*

*Having no connection*
*Not listening*

What else gets in your way?

_____

_____

_____

_____

_____

How motivated do you feel on a scale of 1 (not much), to 10 (very much) to go above and beyond, to do the little things that matter for self and others?

Self: _____

Others: _____

## The evidenced based benefits of engagement to you and compassion

Engagement is very much a big part of compassionate care for healthcare practitioners. Although it can be argued that it takes up too much, truly little time is needed for practitioners to be compassionate with their patients (Trzeciak et al., 2019). This can be done in less than a minute by using compassionate communication to forge a connection with the client. When it comes to having time for patients, it can help to explore Carol Dweck's ideas around mindset. In her work on fixed and growth mindsets, Dweck argues that someone who has a fixed mindset will believe that something cannot be done, while with a growth mindset the person believes that it can. Thinking that we do have time, or we can be available to be compassionate frees us from the negativity holding us back. It also helps to know what it takes to be compassionate at that moment. Brief moments spent with patients are enough to establish a compassionate connection. Healthcare practitioners giving their time and being friendly to patients especially when they see that they are lonely are considered compassionate. Spending time with patients can also help identify issues that might not have been noticed before (Brown-Johnson et al., 2019).

While you may think you have little time for patients, it is often the little things that make the most difference to patients. Patients often speak of the power of small rather than grand gestures that help convey compassion (Bramley & Matiti, 2014). The simple act of holding a patient's hand can be enough to be effective in their suffering (Peters, 2006). The little things that matter to patients are things like playing cards, making tea, and the practitioner having a chat with them (Jack & Tetley, 2016). Similarly, small acts like bringing them their favourite soap, helping them with eating or bathing, and making them feel comfortable, are also perceived as compassionate (Perry, 2009; Hunter et al., 2017).

Despite some nursing students ranking the little things such as fetching a glass of water as the least important for care, patients feel that sometimes these things are what matter most (Hung et al., 2017). Being cared for by a nurse who engages with the patient and attends to the little things like fluffing up a pillow or making them a cup of tea, provides more than just physical care. These acts of compassion have the power to nurture psychological comfort and promote recovery (Kralik et al., 1997).

Studies show that the simple things such as making a cup of tea, taking the patient to the toilet, or holding their hand are reassuring enough to reduce suffering, and be a powerful expression of compassion (Bramley & Matiti, 2014; Hung et al., 2017; Peters, 2006). Practitioners also experience compassion satisfaction by engaging in activities that go beyond their regular duties, showing that the benefits matter to staff as well as patients. These small but significant acts can be considered elements of the art of helping that span further beyond the science. Patients feel compassion from practitioners who go beyond their regular duties (Sinclair et al., 2016). This is seen among physicians' assistants as well as other healthcare staff (Skaff et al., 2003).

## Types of engagement

The different types of engagement identified in this model are having time, doing the little things, and going the extra mile for patients. Each is viewed as an act of compassion. All can bring about great feelings of satisfaction and improve the wellbeing of practitioners and patients.

## Having time for patients

This type of engagement is as simple as it sounds. It is not as much having time but being available for patients. We often hear or tell ourselves that we do not have time, that we are rushed off our feet, or we are jumping from one thing to another and do not have a moment. You will be busy and there will be competing demands that you must contend with but finding the time to spend even some time with patients can be enormously powerful. Your working environment might not always allow you to do this. However, it can be a minute or a few seconds. A lot can be done and happen in that brief period if we know how to make better use of it.

---

### BOX 10.1  HAVING TIME FOR PATIENTS

Things to ask yourself:

*How much time am I spending with patients/clients?*
*What more could I do to be available for them?*

---

You could spend a few minutes chatting with them. Catch up with patients that you have been meaning to speak with to see how they are doing. While you might not be able to do this for all your patients, try and make time for and treat those that you do as your priority. Being available for clients who require your attention can make a massive difference to their experience of therapy or support. Taking time to speak but also notice things about your client or patient can lead to compassion. Time can involve reflection in that moment or after to think about your client and their needs or what you can do for the next time you see them. It can be about not leaving them unattended, especially at times when they are very anxious, say before they are going to enter the theatre or attending therapy for the first time. Asking how their day was, or what has changed since you last spoke are ways to engage the client and break the ice.

## The little things

Intricately linked to making time for patients, doing the little things that matter to clients and patients is another way to express compassion to them. This can be as simple as making them a tea or coffee, fluffing their pillow, or helping them with something such as getting to the toilet or a room if they are lost.

---

### BOX 10.2   THE LITTLE THINGS

Things to ask yourself:

*What are the little things I can do that would help the other?*
*How might they help my client/patient?*

---

This can include giving someone the time and space they need to rest, reflect, and recover. Giving them room to find their words and articulate what they need to say. Introducing yourself and asking if it is okay to enter a room, which is considered polite are expressions of compassion. It can also be about doing things that are personal to them but form a human connection between you both. For example, washing a patient's hair or bathing them. This is especially important if you work in end-of-life care where preparing the patient's body with sensitive care, and respect for the deceased and their family is a profound act of compassion. Advocate for them by supporting them to make that important phone call. Use handouts and notes to share information. Printed material can come in handy later after a session when the client needs a little reminder of the exercises and be useful for them. Talking about the small things in their life that bring much pain can also be a way to express engagement with them.

Bringing them an extra pillow or a cup of tea are ways to express the little things. Staying by their side when they need you most. You might even sing, dance, or bring laughter to them by expressing yourself in ways that show this in a respectful yet light-hearted way. It could be as simple as holding their hand and using supportive compassionate words to reassure them. When a patient is not eating, it can be the little piece of their favourite chocolate that gives them that moment of compassionate care. Equally, getting the little clinical things right can make the difference to the care being delivered. If we get better at these little things, we get better and are more likely to avoid the big things when mistakes are made. These little things can leave patients with an overall positive and compassionate impression of their healthcare experience. They become the important things that matter most and are crucial to compassion and care.

## Going the extra mile (above and beyond)

In some cases, this can mean literally going the extra mile. In rural areas, going the extra mile or few to ensure that the patient is getting the treatment and care they need, means physically driving to them. There are limits to this as practitioners need to be aware of their mental health and wellbeing. Knowing your boundaries will help protect you from going too far. It is about going out of your way for the other person and doing something extra for them.

---

**BOX 10.3  GOING THE EXTRA MILE**

Things to ask yourself:

*What am I doing to go above and beyond my regular duties for this person? In what ways can I do something more for them?*

---

Things you can do to achieve this are, attending a client's art exhibition, and being there out of hours at times when they might need you most. Try to always find a way when there is an emergency.

## Simple exercises – going above and beyond

One nurse I worked with, recalled an elderly patient asking her for a specific bar of soap. The soap held special meaning for the patient, but she was not able to get this due to her being in hospital and not having anyone to get it for her. At the end of her shift, the nurse drove around town until she found the soap. She brought it in for the patient the next day and gave it to her. This seemingly little thing made the patient incredibly happy and was seen as an act of compassion that went above and beyond. While not all of us can go to these lengths, it is an example of what compassionate engagement looks like in practice.

Think of someone you work with, a client or patient and consider what you can do for them to go above and beyond to demonstrate compassion.

_____

_____

_____

_____

_____

## Summary

### Definitions

Engagement is defined as the little things done for patients, going the extra mile to make them feel looked after, and having time for them.

### Key indicators

Having time for patients, small acts, going the extra mile

### Psychology

As engagement is associated with doing things for others it links strongly with the psychology of behaviour.

### Evidenced by

Taking the time to be with patients and engage in small but significant acts of care. Doing the little things such as bringing them a cup of tea or an extra pillow when requested.

### Prevalence of this strength

Engagement can help improve patient wellbeing and is viewed as a compassionate act.

### Reflective questions

_How often do I engage with patients and do the little things for them?_
_What am I currently doing or can do to demonstrate this strength in myself (and others)?_
_What was the last significant thing I did for a client that was beyond my regular duties?_

### Combing strengths

Engagement combines best with connection, communication, and empathy. It can also work with character when you express your kindness to others.

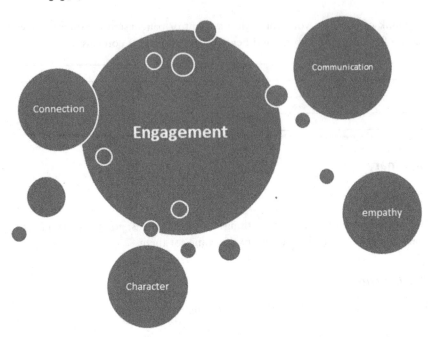

**FIGURE 10.1**  How engagement combines with other compassion strengths

## Conclusion

This chapter has introduced you to the compassion strength of engagement and how doing the little things, going the extra mile, and having time for patients can make a massive difference to their experiences of care. These simple but effective acts allow you to show compassion in new ways that bring compassion satisfaction into your work. That alone should be more than enough reasons to engage more with your patients and give them those little moments of joy that they need and deserve.

What have you learned that you did not know before?

_____

_____

_____

_____

_____

## References

Bramley, L., & Matiti, M. (2014). How does it really feel to be in my shoes? Patients' experiences of compassion within nursing care and their perceptions of developing compassionate nurses. *Journal of Clinical Nursing, 23*, 2790–2799. 10.1111/jocn.12537

Brown-Johnson, C., Schwartz, R., Maitra, A., Haverfield, M. C., Tierney, A., Shaw, J. G., …, & Zulman, D. M. (2019). What is clinician presence? A qualitative interview study comparing physician and non-physician insights about practices of human connection. *BMJ open*, *9*(11), e030831. doi: 10.1136/bmjopen-2019-030831

Henderson, Angela (2001). Emotional labor and nursing: an under-appreciated aspect of caring work. *Nursing Inquiry*, 8, 130–138. 10.1046/j.1440-1800.2001.00097.x

Hung, Lillian, Phinney, Alison, Chaudhury, Habib, Rodney, Paddy, Tabamo, Jenifer, & Bohl, Doris (2017). "Little things matter!" Exploring the perspectives of patients with dementia about the hospital environment. *International Journal of Older People Nursing*, 12, e12153. 10.1111/opn.12153

Hunter, D. J., McCallum, J., & Howes, D. (2017). Doing the little things: the meaning of compassionate care to Scottish student nurses. *Journal of Nursing and Health Care*, 5, 1.

Jack, K. F., & Tetley, J. (2016). Using poems to explore the meaning of compassion to undergraduate nursing students. *International Practice Development Journal*, 6, 1–13.

Keyko, Kacey, Cummings, Greta G., Yonge, Olive, & Wong, Carol A. (2016). Work engagement in professional nursing practice: A systematic review. *International Journal of Nursing Studies*, 61, 142–164. 10.1016/j.ijnurstu.2016.06.003.

Kralik, Debbie, Koch, Tina, & Wotton, Karen (1997). Engagement and detachment: understanding patients' experiences with nursing. *Journal of Advanced Nursing*, 26, 399–407. 10.1046/j.1365-2648.1997.1997026399.x.

Perry, B. (2009). Conveying compassion through attention to the essential ordinary. *Nursing Older People*, 21, 6 10.7748/nop2009.07.21.6.14.c7137.

Peters, M. A. (2006). Compassion: an investigation into the experience of nursing faculty. *International Journal of Human Caring*, 10, 38–46. 10.20467/1091-5710.10.3.38

Raper, James L. (2014). Going the Extra Mile for Retention and Re-engagement in Care: Nurses Make a Difference. *Journal of the Association of Nurses in AIDS Care*, 25, 108–111. 10.1016/j.jana.2013.10.002

Sinclair, Shane, Norris, Jill M., McConnell, Shelagh J., Chochinov, Harvey Max, Hack, Thomas F., Hagen, Neil A., McClement, Susan, & Bouchal, Shelley Raffin (2016). Compassion: a scoping review of the healthcare literature. *BMC Palliative Care*, 15 10.1186/s12904-016-0080-0.

Skaff, K. O., Toumey, C. P., Rapp, D., & Fahringer, D. (2003). *Measuring compassion in physician assistants. JAAPA-Journal of the American Academy of Physicians Assistants*, 16, 31–38.

Spence Laschinger, Heather K., Leiter, Michael, Day, Arla, & Gilin, Debra (2009). Workplace empowerment, incivility, and burnout: impact on staff nurse recruitment and retention outcomes. *Journal of Nursing Management*, 17, 302–311. 10.1111/j.1365-2 834.2009.00999.x.

Trzeciak, S., Mazzarelli, A., & Booker, C. (2019). *Compassionomics: The revolutionary scientific evidence that caring makes a difference*, 287–319.

# 11

# INTERPERSONAL SKILLS

## Introduction

In this chapter, we will focus on the interpersonal skills that healthcare staff and students need to develop their compassion strengths. Working in healthcare environments means that students and practitioners will interact with others daily. The patient–professional interaction is a key element of the therapeutic process and is critical to the quality of care received. Interpersonal skills can help achieve the connection between patient and practitioner. In this chapter you will learn:

1. What we mean by interpersonal skills
2. The opposites of interpersonal skills
3. Why we need interpersonal skills
4. The obstacles to this compassion strength
5. The types of interpersonal skills

## What are interpersonal skills?

Interpersonal skills refer to the aptitude someone has that enables them to interact with others and form productive relationships. Someone with effective interpersonal skills can communicate with different people at all levels and from various backgrounds. Psychology can tell us a great deal about ourselves and other people. For instance, there are different dynamics at play when we communicate and interact with others. For instance, Transactional Analysis (TA) tells us that we can be speaking to a parent, adult, or child and that we might also adopt this way of communicating with them (Berne, 1968). The goal is to become more aware of our communication style and speak

DOI: 10.4324/9781003276425-11

appropritaley to those we are speaking to. This applies to the healthcare setting just as much as it does in our everyday interactions. Communication and interpersonal skills are often grouped as one when in fact they are two distinct strengths of compassion. Whereas communication relates to how practitioners speak, listen, and express themselves through body language, interpersonal skills are used to build a therapeutic relationship, collect, and relay important information, create flexibility, and ensure that the patient and healthcare team understand one another. They are how people can manage interpersonal relationships using a variety of skills with communication being core to how they interact with others.

## The opposite of compassionate interpersonal skills

One opposite to interpersonal skills is intrapersonal skills. While the two may sound the same, one is concerned with other people and the other with the self. Although this is not necessarily a terrible thing it does mean that a person's attention is turned inward to the self, rather than outward to the people around them. This can serve a purpose that is helpful when being reflective and developing the self. It is concerned with knowing the self, resilience, and self-regulation. Another opposite is impersonal. Not having the ability to relate to others and productively collaborate with them.

## Obstacles to this strength

*Lack of empathy*
*Little thought or understanding of others*
*Inability to connect*
*No self-awareness or insight*
*Struggle to communicate information in a compassionate way*
*Not involving the client or patient in their care*
*Confusion amongst the team*
*Poor negotiation or conflict management skills*
*Unresolved personal issues*
*Lack of boundaries*
*Negative self-esteem and self-talk*

What else gets in your way?

_____

_____

_____

_____

_____

How motivated do you feel on a scale of 1 (not much), to 10 (very much) to use your interpersonal skills?

_____

_____

_____

_____

_____

## Why interpersonal skills are needed for practice?

Effective interpersonal skills rely not only on effective communication but on the practitioner to adapt their behaviour to the context, situation, environmental, cultural, and psychological needs of the person and achieve prosocial goals (Rubin & Martin, 1994). These skills enable cooperation between not only the client and therapists but the whole team involved in the care of the patient. Managers can help their staff grow and learn by using their interpersonal skills. They are especially helpful when collecting and sharing information between staff. Interpersonal skills such as self-awareness can help individuals identify any unconscious biases or negative stereotypes they might have towards certain groups which may be preventing practitioners from understanding or treating them with compassion. They can help with co-worker communication and when making the patient part of their care.

Core competencies of all healthcare workers include interpersonal skills. They include the effective practice of communication, empathy, and connection skills to communicate with patients, their families, colleagues, and other health professionals (Wysong & Driver, 2009). Interpersonal skills are often mistaken for communication skills, when in fact they are not mutually exclusive. Peplau's (1991) theory of interpersonal relations emphasises the relevance of interpersonal skills in nursing. Good patient-practitioner interactions are associated with multiple benefits such as treatment success (Mauksch et al., 2008), and patient satisfaction. They are also linked to the wide range of medical consultation times globally which differs between countries (Irving et al., 2017). Effective interpersonal skills can improve the quality of the interaction during the consultation regardless of the time spent with patients (Bellier et al., 2022). When one shows good interpersonal skills to others, they also provide an example of a trustworthy individual to clients who may not have had that in their life. Usually, if someone has not, they will act in ways that can be perceived as 'difficult.'

For good reasons they will have demands and wants that will take you away from your work while you try to address their concerns. Interpersonal skills can help you navigate this and create solutions for problems between more than one person. Interpersonal skills such as self-awareness can assist in the management of conflict between people in the healthcare system. Patients, colleagues, and family members can all become highly charged when under immense stress. Learning and developing interpersonal skills can therefore help students and practitioners understand themselves and the people they treat on a deeper level (Gjestvang et al., 2021).

Interpersonal skills are critical for understanding and treating people with communication issues. Adapting communication so that information is delivered in an understandable way leads to a greater experience for the carer and patient. They can be used when approaching difficult conversations with compassion. For example, when combined with communication it can help to communicate better in situations that are tense or emotional such as breaking bad news.

Interpersonal skills can be used to bring patients into their care. To promote effective patient care it is vital that patients are included in the process and can make decisions on their own. Practitioner and patient working together on a management plan that considers past experiences and the patient's needs is helpful (Pinto, 2012). Taking a more active role in their care can empower patients and lead to more positive health outcomes. For example, CBT is an effective form of therapy based on shared decision-making and empowerment.

## The evidenced based benefits of interpersonal skills for compassion

Interpersonal skills can be used alongside other compassion strengths such as empathy, connection, and communication, to build and maintain close relationships with clients, patients, and colleagues, as well as help, manage conflict if it arises. It is important and helpful for all involved in the care of others to develop strong collegial relationships that help the client or patient. Watson (2011) defined caring as a significant moral and ethical guide that represented the values of empathy, communication, competency, and interpersonal skills, using such words as compassion, joy, hope, openness, love, and peace to reflect the connection between the physical and spiritual worlds of patient and nurse (Jesse & Alligood, 2013). The continued development of clinical, communication, empathic and interpersonal skills help ensure that practitioners can deliver compassion to their patients. Providing compassionate care for patients includes attending to the needs of the family, as well as communicating with other healthcare colleagues. As such this requires the use of interpersonal skills. Working together with and involving patients and their families during the care process is often considered to be an effective expression of compassion (Kneafsey et al., 2015). The ability to explain clinical symptoms to patients and their families reassures them of what each procedure meant, and what they should expect from care. The importance of interpersonal skills relates to making informed choices and is also recognised by registered nurses and nursing students as behaving honestly and professionally (Durkin et al., 2019). Therapists can work on their interpersonal skills to help foster a greater working therapeutic alliance with their clients. For Rogers (1957), this involves genuineness, unconditional acceptance, and empathy for the client.

## Types of interpersonal skills

There are several different types of interpersonal skills that students and practitioners can develop through education and on-the-job training/experience with patients. The key interpersonal skills associated with compassion across healthcare professions are, collecting and sharing information, self-awareness, and involving the patient in their care. Granted, some will focus more on one or two depending on the professions. For example, to empower their clients, a therapist or psychologist is more likely to engage them in their care. Here we will look at each in more detail and explore ways in which they can be developed.

## Collecting and sharing information

Collecting and sharing information is central to all healthcare professions. It is the way practitioners get to know more about their clients and patients and how they translate back to them what is happening to them. This can range from collecting personal information to sharing good or unwelcome news with a client and their loved ones. This must be done with compassion.

---

### BOX 11.1   COLLECTING AND SHARING INFORMATION

Things to ask yourself:

*When asking questions do I speak clearly in a way that the person understands me? How often do I use medical jargon when speaking with others?*

---

To do this, avoid jargon and talk in understandable terms. Check that they understand what you are saying to them, especially when describing a technical or clinical procedure. Encourage them to ask questions so that they are clear about what is happening or going to happen. Using open questions rather than closed ones adds to the clarity of the questions asked. Be enthusiastic and interested in the client when collecting information but not intrusive.

---

### BOX 11.2   UNDERSTANDABLE LANGUAGE

Things to ask yourself:

*Can I translate medical and clinical terms into understandable language for my patients and their families?*

---

Translating medical terms in such a way that the patient or client and their family understand what is happening to them. Providing information.

## Self-awareness

This type of interpersonal skill can be defined as one's conscious knowledge of character, motivations, feelings, and desires. It relates to unconscious biases or negative stereotypes towards other people and groups. Being aware of this can release any blockages that might occur when caring for another person. Sometimes something will bug you about a person and you might not be able to figure out what it is or why they have that effect on you. Self-awareness is great for identifying what it could be and not letting it take control. Self-disclosure is linked to this too. You might be aware of how anxious you become in certain situations. Building your distress tolerance can help with this. This is a lack of anxiety in social environments and around uncomfortable situations. It is also associated with the ability to receive criticism from others.

---

### BOX 11.3  SELF-AWARENESS

Things to ask yourself:

*How self-aware are you of your own biases?*
*What negative stereotypes do you hold?*
*How open are you with others?*
*What situations or stories make you feel anxious?*
*How flexible am I in my work?*
*How much of a team player am I?*

---

Mindfulness is an effective way to develop self-awareness. Simply being mindful of your thoughts and feelings when they arise can make you more self-aware. Accepting whatever is happening at that moment increases self-awareness of pain, anger, frustration, or judgement. This increased self-awareness can help practitioners decide how they will respond to situations more positively in which they find themselves holding onto negative biases. It can also help if they are experiencing any feelings of distress. By being more accepting, they create more tolerance and compassion for themselves and others and are better able to manage conflicts or difficult conversations.

## Simple exercise – journaling

An effective way to become more self-aware of how you relate to others is through journaling. Writing down your thoughts and feelings about yourself and others is a fantastic way to see what might be behind your blocks and behaviours towards others. Being honest with yourself can help set you free of them and move forward with compassion. Reflection is a process of experimental learning.

## Engaging clients and patients in their care

Research shows that when patients are included in their care, they feel treated with compassion. This can be very empowering for them, changing the dynamic between the clinician and patient from one that is one-sided to an equal level.

---

**BOX 11.4  ENGAGING CLIENTS AND PATIENTS IN THEIR CARE**

Things to ask yourself:

*How often do you show an interest in your clients' ideas about their health?*
*How often do you involve your patient in the decision-making process?*

---

Taking an interest in your patient's ideas about their health and allowing them to be more informed in their care is a compassionate interpersonal skill. Give as much information as the client or patient wants about their situation and involve them in decisions during their time with you. Where possible bring them into the decision-making process. Motivating your clients, patients, and your colleagues. Believe in them even when they find it hard to do themselves.

## Summary

### Definitions

The use of other strengths such as communication and connection to alleviate patients' stress and worries, and to communicate with patients and colleagues on various levels.

### Key indicators

Involving patient and their families, Communication with colleagues, Knowledge of clinical terms

## Psychology

This compassion strength covers the behaviours and cognitions associated with being compassionate. For example, using cognitive abilities to translate clinical terms to patients and vice versa when communicating a patient's needs to other members of the care team.

## Evidenced by

Use of skills to relate, and connect to the patient, family members, colleagues, and all involved in the care of patients. Ability to explain medical terms and communicate what is going on throughout the care journey.

## Prevalence of this strength

The ability to speak to people on different levels from the bed to the head is a highly sought-after compassion strength.

## Reflective questions

*What am I currently doing or can do to demonstrate this strength in myself (and others)? What do I find most difficult when communicating with patients, their families, and colleagues?*

## Combing strengths

Of course, one of the most obvious ways to combine interpersonal strengths is with communication. This can help when talking to different people involved in your practice. Interpersonal skills work well with empathy and connection too.

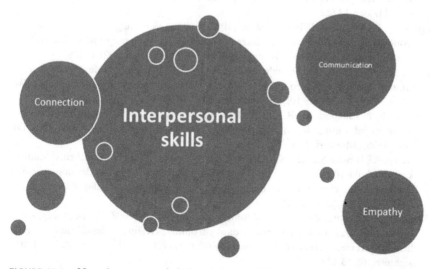

**FIGURE 11.1**  How interpersonal skills combines with other compassion strengths

## Conclusion

In this chapter, we have explored how interpersonal skills can be used as a compassion strength. Looking at the different types, you should now have some insight into the various ways you can utilise your skills in your profession. They can be used with other compassion strengths to reach your clients and speak to them in ways that they understand so that the goals of care and compassion can be achieved.

What have you learned that you did not know before?

_____

_____

_____

_____

_____

## References

Bellier, Alexandre, Labarère, José, Putkaradze, Zaza, Cavalie, Guillaume, Carras, Sylvain, Pelen, Félix, Paris, Adeline, & Chaffanjon, Philippe (2022). Effectiveness of a multi-faceted intervention to improve interpersonal skills of physicians in medical consultations (EPECREM): protocol for a randomised controlled trial. BMJ Open, 12, e051600 10.1136/bmjopen-2021-051600

Berne Eric Dr PhD (1973). Transcription of Eric Berne in Vienna, 1968. Transactional Analysis Bulletin, 3, 63–72. 10.1177/036215377300300117

Bray, Lucy, O'Brien, Mary R., Kirton, Jennifer, Zubairu, Kate, & Christiansen, Angela (2014). The role of professional education in developing compassionate practitioners: A mixed methods study exploring the perceptions xof health professionals and pre-registration students. Nurse Education Today, 34, 480–486. 10.1016/j.nedt.2013.06.017

Durkin, J., Usher, K., & Jackson, D. (2019). Embodying compassion: A systematic review of the views of nurses and patients. _Journal of clinical nursing, 28_(9–10), 1380–1392. 10.1111/jocn.14722

Gjestvang, B., Kvigne, K. J., Hoel, E., & Kvaal, K. S. (2021). A training course on interpersonal relationships using role play in a Master of Mental Health Care programme–The students' experiences. _Nurse Education Today, 102,_ 104887. 10.1016/j.nedt.2021.104887

Irving, G., Neves, A. L., Dambha-Miller, H., et al (2017). International variations in primary care physician consultation time: a systematic review of 67 countries. _BMJ Open, 7,_ e017902. doi: 10.1136/bmjopen-2017-017902

Jesse, D. E. & Alligood, M. R. (2013). Jean Watson: Watson's Philosophy and theory of transpersonal caring. In M. R. Alligood, _Nursing theorists and their work_ (8th Ed, pp. 79–98). Missouri: Elsevier.

Kneafsey, R., Brown, S., Sein, K., Chamley, C., & Parsons, J. (2015). A qualitative study of key stakeholders' perspectives on compassion in healthcare and the development of a framework for compassionate interpersonal relations. _Journal of Clinical Nursing, 25,_ 70–79. 10.1111/jocn.12964

Mauksch, L. B., Dugdale, D. C., Dodson, S., & Epstein, R. (2008). Relationship, communication, and efficiency in the medical encounter: creating a clinical model from a literature review. _Archives of internal medicine, 168_(13), 1387–1395. doi:10.1001/archinte.168.13.1387

Peplau, H. E. (1991). *Interpersonal relations in nursing: A conceptual frame of reference for psychodynamic nursing.* London: Springer Publishing Company.

Pinto, R. Z., Ferreira, M. L., Oliveira, V. C., Franco, M. R., Adams, R., Maher, C. G., & Ferreira, P. H. (2012). Patient-centred communication is associated with positive therapeutic alliance: a systematic review. *Journal of physiotherapy, 58*(2), 77–87. 10.1016/S1836-9553(12)70087-5

Rogers, C. R. (1957). The necessary and sufficient conditions of therapeutic personality change. *Journal of Consulting Psychology, 21*(2), 95–103. 10.1037/h0045357

Rubin, R. B., & Martin, M. M. (1994). Development of a measure of interpersonal communication competence. *Communication Research Reports, 11*(1), 33–44. 10.1080/08824099409359938

Watson, J. (2011). *Human caring science.* Sudbury, MA: Jones & Bartlett Publishers.

Wysong, P. R., & Driver, E. (2009). Patients' perceptions of nurses' skill. *Critical Care Nurse, 29*(4), 24–37. doi: 10.4037/ccn2009241

# 12

# COMPETENCE

## Introduction

This chapter focuses on the competencies that can help you when showing your compassion strengths. While the harder skills of clinical competence are given priority over softer skills of compassion in all healthcare roles, there is no reason to say that clinical skills are harder ways of showing compassion. The clinical skills that practitioners use to alleviate the suffering of their clients, create the same if not stronger outcomes for them concerning their healthcare needs. As you read this chapter you will discover the main competencies that overlap between professions and can be used to show compassion strengths. I have tried to unify them the best I can to make them applicable to all or as many healthcare professions as possible. Knowing what competencies are needed for your professions, can help identify what you need to develop the skills that will allow you to perform your work, and be compassionate. In this chapter you will learn:

1. What we mean by competence
2. The opposites of competence
3. Why we need competence
4. The obstacles to this compassion strengths
5. The types of competence

## What is competence?

Competence refers to the underlying characteristics that a person demonstrates in their work (Boyatzis, 1982). It includes a set of **traits, skills, abilities, and knowledge** that helps them achieve best performance in their chosen field. Their purpose is to ensure that care is delivered safely and with high-quality outcomes to

DOI: 10.4324/9781003276425-12

individuals and groups (Langins & Borgermans, 2016). The knowledge aspect involves knowing the procedures, and information to do with their subject area that is about the work. This can include facts and procedures or techniques that can be used to support someone physically or psychologically. Traits are the personal aspects of the individual that enable them to do their job in a way that they respond correctly. So, for instance, compassionate character traits would be suitable in helping professions over colder traits. Abilities are the things that have been learned through experience and that which the professional brings with them to practice and contribute to other areas of competency. Skills refer to the practitioner using their knowledge and understanding to apply this effectively with their clients and patients through either cognitive, motor, or social skills (Handel, 2003).

## The opposite of clinical competence

When someone lacks clinical competence, they show an inability to perform their duties effectively. Clinical incompetence is the clearest way the describe this. It can lead to mistakes in care, as well as increase the client's and their family's anxiety and worry. When burned out it can be easy to forget the practical skills or replace compassion for complete competence. Certain practitioners may lack professional growth, while others simply have not progressed to the next stage of their career development, thus limiting their knowledge and ability.

## Why clinical competence is important for practice

Clinical competence helps you understand the clinical needs of your patient or clients so that you can deliver the right treatment for them. To be clinically competent, practitioners are expected to be able to apply their skills and abilities to new experiences as well as more familiar procedures. According to Benner (1982), healthcare workers acquire their competence over time, transitioning from novice to expert through several stages during their career. Students with little or no training are considered novices who after training, clinical experience, and professional growth, become more an expert in their field. Similar models have been developed for clinical psychology that transition from novice to expert. The student goes from novice to advanced beginner, competence, proficiency, and expertise (Sharpless & Barber, 2009). These competencies can range from generic skills to more specific. Yet, clinical competence is not to be confused with an absolute end goal. It is a continuously evolving dynamic process for the individual that changes and renews itself throughout the lifetime of their career. Healthcare professionals move from abstract knowledge to the application of concrete clinical practice developed through various stages of experience and interactions with clients and patients. Equally, not all will follow a linear path toward reaching what can be described as competence in their chosen craft. Not everyone moves across each stage in the same order.

Before they can become registered, practitioners must meet the standards for competency and must maintain these standards throughout their career for their respected field. This ensures that they have the knowledge and skills to effectively complete the clinical duties underpinning their work. It also helps safeguard the patient and protect practitioners from the threat of malpractice. This is the same for therapists, psychologists, social workers, physicians, midwives, and all other healthcare students and professionals.

To be clinically competent in your work is considered more important to the welfare of the people you care for. Practitioners need to have the skills and abilities to deliver treatment to expected results. They have a responsibility to their clients and patients to be up to date with the clinical procedures, and trained in the skills of their trade, to enable safe and effective treatment. Safety is of paramount importance for all that are treated by their practitioner. Having the skills to do your job to a high standard can be the difference between life and death.

A wider range of skills increases the practitioner's helping repertoire. When you develop your skills, you become more knowledgeable. Using this knowledge and gaining valuable experience makes you more of an expert in your field. Evidence-based care is at the forefront of healthcare strategies. The practitioner's technical skills such as providing medication, and being available when in pain, help to improve the well-being of patients (Ortega-Galán et al., 2019). There are initiatives to make care better for the patient and clients that use the service. But despite the need to achieve targets for improving the care experience compassion can sometimes be forgotten about. Regarding adherence to following correct procedures, care and treatment interventions must be delivered with competence. This helps avoid doing the right things badly or the wrong things well, when what matters most is that practitioners do the right things well and to acceptable standards (Fairburn & Cooper, 2011). Yet, evidence shows that competence and compassion complement each other, and lead to greater outcomes for patients and practitioners.

## Obstacles to clinical competence

*Lack of training*
*Inappropriate education*
*Not covered by a governing body*
*Not making use of continuous professional development*
*Poor use of skills and abilities*
*A wrong attitude towards people*
*Lack of support from the organisation to develop skills*
*Unprofessional behavior*

What other things get in your way?

_____

_____

_____

_____

_____

How motivated do you feel on a scale of 1 (not much), to 10 (very much) by your competency skills?

_____

_____

_____

_____

_____

## The evidenced based benefits of clinical competence for compassion

How is competence a compassion strength? While competence is often seen as being separate from compassion, research shows that it is very much a part of being compassionate (Durkin, 2019; 2020). We hear about compassion competency where practitioners are competent in their ability to be compassionate. However, taking a different view this book sees clinical competence as part of being compassionate. If we think back to the definition of compassion, which is to alleviate suffering, then it makes sense that being clinically competent to do the work that eases pain, reduces suffering, and attends to clinical needs, is an act of compassion. When students and practitioners are competent in their clinical skills, they spend less worrying about doing the job properly and focus on being compassionate.

There are arguments on both sides for why both are fundamental to compassionate care. Clinically competent care can leave clients and patients feeling empty and de-humanised, while compassion alone does not help patients heal or get better. Therefore, both are needed for true holistic care and the desired outcomes for patients and practitioners. Compassion requires more than the awareness of suffering, just like care relies on more than clinical competence. Practitioners need to demonstrate the intelligence and skills of their profession as well as other core compassion strengths to ensure that patients and clients are treated as people and not just a condition. For person-centered compassionate care to be realised competence must align with compassion and vice versa (Lown et al., 2011; Sharp et al., 2016).

Even though compassion and competence are key to care, both require judgement from the practitioner about when to use them and in what situation. In most cases, patients and clients would take competence over compassion. This can depend on the nature of their treatment. For example, if someone is going for surgery, they would want the surgeon to show their clinical competence to perform the surgery. If there was a complication or delay in getting to the theatre, then a compassionate approach using communication and empathy would be needed to reassure the patient of this. Both are equally powerful ways that the practitioner can alleviate physical and psychological suffering. This tells us that competence is an act of compassion just not in the classic form that we usually associate with compassionate practice. It is more an example of compassionate behaviour than the traditionally associated emotional response. To elaborate on this, here is an example for you to consider.

Surgeons are often criticised for lacking compassion. However, if you need surgery to fix a broken bone or life-saving brain surgery, then you are suffering and the only way to relieve this is through clinical skills and competence of the surgeon and their team. This detachment from the human emotional element of the patient is what makes the surgeon good at what they do when conducting an operation. In times of stress when quick thinking trumps emotion, I know which one I would prefer in this situation.

At the same time, the importance of both these abilities should not be underestimated in the context of compassionate care. There is evidence to show that practitioners who are perceived to be more compassionate are also considered to be more competent (Heinze et al., 2020). The unique interplay between the two shows just how the clinical skills demonstrated by healthcare students and staff are and can be thought of as a strength of a compassionate practitioner.

Technical skills can support people through each stage of their treatment and can be used to control symptoms and address needs throughout the patient/client journey. Such competence is a necessity for all who access care. They should be used alongside other compassion strengths to reduce pain, the intensity of suffering, and anxiety and improve overall wellbeing. Competency helps the practitioner find the most suitable interventions that will support clients through the experiences and alleviate suffering. It also helps improve quality of life.

Clinical competence becomes compassionate when all staff knows what they are doing and perform their duties with confidence (Badger & Royse, 2012). Being competent in evidence and knowledge-based practice is how practitioners can help patients' (Tehranineshat et al., 2018). This includes an understanding of professional boundaries (Lee & Seomun, 2016) and using that awareness to allow patients to take responsibility for their own lives. A feature of boundaries includes advocacy in the practitioner's role, where this act offers strength to the patient, and compassion can be viewed as celebrating a patient's accomplishment. Therapists' competence refers to the clinical judgement of the therapist and the range of conditions they can work with to meet their clients' goals through different interventions. Therapists require competencies such as therapeutic alliance to enable the delivery of therapeutic skills and create a sense of safety for clients, knowledge, and understanding to inform all other competencies and use of supervision to grow and develop skills (Liddell et al., 2017).

As certain nations become more ethnically diverse, there is a need to include the cultural competencies needed when providing care for patients from multicultural backgrounds (Betancourt et al., 2002). This helps to integrate the cultural needs of patients and raise nursing students' self-awareness (Campinha-Bacote, 2002).

## Types of competence

Different competencies apply to each of the healthcare professions. These can vary from novice to expert depending on their education and experience. While there are distinct differences between professions such as nurses' competencies and therapists, here I have tried to bring together a few of the core elements into four core overarching domains that demonstrate a unified understanding of clinical competency concerning compassion. All have the aim of attending to the patient's needs, alleviating their suffering, and improving wellbeing. They align to become a competent practitioner who evolves from a novice to expert, including the traits, skills, abilities, and attitude needed to develop into competent healthcare professional. It can help to look at each one to identify your training and competency needs. They are:

## Clinical knowledge and treatment application/research and evidenced based practice or evidence informed practice

First, for any student or practicing healthcare professional, clinical knowledge is key to providing compassionate care. This type of competence relates to the practitioner's ability to understand clinical and scientific knowledge and apply it to practice. Knowing what treatment approach works for each patient or the best therapeutic intervention for clients means that you can give them the best care possible. Indeed, those taking their first steps into education and practice will have limited knowledge and application time in this area. They will learn through a mixture of education and practice in clinical placements. Others with more experience will have gained insight into the basics but still have space to learn more. Evidenced based practice is the cornerstone of all healthcare professions.

---

### BOX 12.1   EVIDENCE BASED PRACTICE

Things to ask yourself:

*What clinical knowledge do I have at this present moment?*
*How is this helping me become competent in my field?*
*How informed am I of new evidence in my area of expertise?*

---

Think about how you demonstrate clinical judgement. How do you become competent at what you do? If your job requires you to diagnose, what do you base this on? What evidence do you have to support the practice you use? For example, if you are suggesting to a client that a certain type of therapy is going to work for them, what do you base this on? These kinds of questions must be considered before any intervention. Equally, if you are collaborating with patients and want to suggest a treatment, being informed of the recent and strongest evidence to support it, can help you make clinically sound research-informed choices. It would be helpful to keep up to date with recent developments in practice so that you are informed of what is new and can be applied to your work.

## Provide patient cantered care in relation to psychosocial and cultural factors

In addition to the prevention of disease, and illness, competence is also about prosocial behaviours that improve wellbeing. Having a greater awareness of the wider picture and the implications of the patient's background are imperative to providing person-cantered care. This is achieved using the other compassion strengths such as character, communication, connection, and engagement. Patient-cantered care puts the person central to the care they receive. It sees them as a unique individual who is worthy of respect, care, and compassion regardless of their background. Having an awareness of diversity can improve your knowledge and understanding of clients and provide a contextual frame for their problems.

---

### BOX 12.2 PSYCHOSOCIAL AND CULTURAL FACTORS

Things to ask yourself:

*What other psychosocial and cultural factors do I need to be aware of about my patient or client?*
*How can this knowledge help me with the people I work with?*

---

How can you use the compassion strength connection to get to understand your patient? In what ways can you use their narrative to combine your clinical knowledge with their world of experience to produce a mutually agreeable solution to the issues they face. No doubt there will be complex interactions of causal factors that have contributed to this that need to be heard and explored without judgement. Work, social, and economic conditions can all contribute to health, both at the individual and global levels. People may feel disadvantaged by their current situation. Childhood living conditions such as poverty or abuse can severely affect their health and wellbeing. Equally, someone with more wealth who can afford adventure holidays in the sun will be at risk of other potential health issues. Gaining insight into this can aid you in helping to understand the patient and provide care that fits in with their holistic needs.

## Practice professionally/professionalism

This type of competence relates to how practitioners behave and act. It refers to how their professional attitude is expressed through interactions with others and the observable behaviours of students and staff. It is how you express yourself as a healthcare professional. They are expected to adhere to ethical guidelines and treat patients and their families as well as colleagues effectively. It is also associated with professional identity and how one comports themselves in different contexts and environments. Doing what is expected of a professional can make them act more like a professional. Attitudes towards the professions, the people you work with, those who use your service, and learning are all key to professionalism. Showing enthusiasm and respect by turning up on time, not being hung over, how you present yourself, your uniform, being respectful to patients, colleague educators demonstrate your professionalism. It is everyone's responsibility to act professionally. This sets the bar for students to emulate when they first encounter practice.

---

### BOX 12.3  PRACTICE PROFESSIONALLY/PROFESSIONALISM

Things to ask yourself:

*How am I acting like a professional in my practice and outside of it?*
*What makes me professional in my field?*

---

Ways in which you can develop your professionalism are through education and on-the-job training, interactions with patients and colleagues, or role modelling someone who embodies the professionalism you look to emulate. This can be someone you work with or in the media. Things like time keeping and working towards appointments are other key features of professional behaviour that show value and respect to the people you treat and the organisation you work for. Good patient care. Are you up to date with the ethical guidelines of your work, do you, know them, follow them, and apply them to your practice depending on what stage of your career you are at? However, professionalism is much more than this. You must also think about how you present yourself outside of work, how you would behave in public, and if you bumped into one of your clients.

## Work in multidisciplinary teams

Multidisciplinary teamwork is described as the collaborative work between healthcare professionals from various backgrounds such as nurses, psychologists, social workers, psychiatrists, doctors, midwives, and social workers. Each profession comes together to combine its skills toward the same collective aim of providing high-quality care (Hogston & Marjoram, 2007). Certain aspects of each person's role will feed into the other, with for example community nurses providing advice on housing just like a social worker would. Knowing and identifying others in the wider team that is or can be part of your case. Colleagues who have specialisms that contribute to your own that when combined provide holistic care for your patient. This might not always apply to your practice, especially if you are a therapist working in your private practice. However, there are still people in the wider community whose knowledge you can draw on to develop that extra level of competency. Working with others helps broaden your knowledge and understanding which when combined brings better outcomes for service users.

---

**BOX 12.4   WORK IN MULTIDISCIPLINARY TEAMS**

Things to ask yourself:

*Who can I learn from in my team?*
*What are the benefits of working in a multidisciplinary team?*
*What do I contribute to the team?*

---

Most healthcare professionals work in multidisciplinary teams. Thinking of the ways you can benefit from this and develop your abilities can help you become more proficient and provide a more holistic approach to patient care. Here other strengths such as communication and interpersonal skills are vital for the delivery of compassionate patient centred care. Developing open communication within your team and between others in and outside of your organisation can ensure that all are aware of clients' and patients' care needs. Consider your contribution and what skills you bring that set you apart but bring wholeness to the care team. What are the ways you can bridge the gaps between yourself, the team, and other professionals? What are the different views you have about treatment that need to be seen as one? For example, a psychiatrist might want to diagnose and prescribe medication to treat a service user, while a psychologist would consider the person's subjective experiences that have led to their mental health condition. Both are called for however, one or both could be more important at those initial stages of the care process. The service user view is also needed. How can you work together and with others to create effective patient care that covers all the patient's needs? To aid with this, using terms such as, we, they, over I and them, creates a team mentality.

## Continued professional development/learning (CPD/L)

This refers to the practitioner being responsible for their learning and professional development. It is how they develop the skills needed to improve their craft and help them succeed in their work. Developments in research and practice evolve quite quickly so it is important to keep up to date. This type of competency requires reflective practice and for the student or practitioner to continuously reflect on their performance both personally and with a mentor, supervisor, or another senior member of staff.

---

**BOX 12.5  CONTINUED PROFESSIONAL DEVELOPMENT/ LEARNING**

Things to ask yourself:

*Where would I place myself on a scale of novice to expert?*
*What learning or training do I need right now?*
*How do I take feedback or criticism about my work?*
*What do I not know?*

---

Regardless of what stage of development you are at, reflecting on your practice can help you find the skills you need to improve to both maintain and improve your overall competencies. There is no shame in admitting you do not know something. An effective way to do this is to keep a journal or log. Writing things down can help you can see what the gaps are in your knowledge and give you a platform to work from. Some professions require you to do this regularly and provide the means to do it in the form of a document. There will always be something new that you can learn, such as a new course that will build your skills repertoire and increase your knowledge. Nevertheless, you as a practitioner must embrace new learning opportunities to improve your knowledge-based skills. It is a personal responsibility and a professional expectation for all. Things you can do to engage in CPD are attending conferences, exploring the research efficacy of interventions, and speaking with colleagues and service users to see how effective or useful something might be for your practice. What professional and academic knowledge do you need to boost your skills?

## Simple exercise – self-check-in

What competencies do I have already?

_____

_____

_____

_____

_____

What do I need to do now to achieve the next level of competence for my role?

_____

_____

_____

_____

_____

What steps will I take to achieve this? (You might want to use SMART goals to help you)

_____

_____

_____

_____

_____

## Summary

### Definitions

Clinical competence is defined as understanding the specialised knowledge and evidence-based care that was needed to do the job proficiently. In doing so the healthcare student and practitioner release cognitive energy spent on thinking about the task at hand, for compassion.

### Key indicators

Professional competence, Skills to do the clinical work.

### Psychology

Clinical competence is demonstrated in the behaviours displayed in practice and cognitive abilities when learning the skills of your profession.

### Evidenced by

Demonstrates confidence in the ability to demonstrate clinical skills competently. Active in continued professional development.

### Prevalence of this strength

Being a competent practitioner is paramount for all healthcare professions. It is found in guidelines and policies and is a core feature of professional development.

## Reflective questions

*What am I currently doing or can do to demonstrate this strength in myself (and others)?*
*How can I develop my professional skills?*
*What skills am I most confident in?*
*Are there any areas that I would like to build upon?*

## Combing strengths

**Competence** works best with interpersonal skills, communication, empathy, and connection. You can use engagement to address the smaller clinical needs of the client or patient.

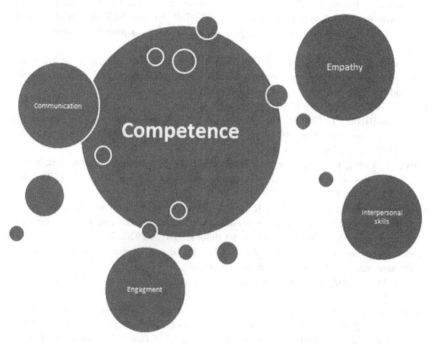

**FIGURE 12.1**  How competence combines with other compassion strengths

## Conclusion

In this chapter, we have covered what competence is and how it relates to compassion. While it may seem that the two are separate, the topics covered, and examples given will hopefully change your mind and shape your thinking and practice in alignment with these ideas. Competence is a strength of compassion that all students and practitioners will have at various stages of their careers. It is recommended that you learn new skills and continue your professional development in ways that complement your compassion to enable you to flourish as a competent and compassionate practitioner.

What have you learned that you did not know before?

_____

_____

_____

_____

_____

## References

Badger, K., & Royse, D. (2012). Describing compassionate care: the burn survivor's perspective. *Journal of Burn Care & Research, 33*, 772–780. 10.1097/BCR.0b013e318254d30b

Benner, P. (1982). From novice to expert. *AJN The American Journal of Nursing, 82*(3), 402–407.

Betancourt, J. R., Green, A. R., & Carrillo, J. E. (2002). *Cultural competence in health care: emerging frameworks and practical approaches* (Vol. 576). New York, NY: Commonwealth Fund, Quality of Care for Underserved Populations.

Boyatzis, R.E. (1982). *The Competent Manager*, Wiley.

Campinha-Bacote, J. (2002). The process of cultural competence in the delivery of healthcare services: A model of care. *Journal of Transcultural Nursing, 13*(3), 181–184. 10.1177%2F10459602013003003

Durkin, J., Usher, K., & Jackson, D. (2019). Embodying compassion: A systematic review of the views of nurses and patients. *Journal of Clinical Nursing, 28*(9–10), 1380–1392. 10.1111/jocn.14722

Durkin, J., Jackson, D., & Usher, K. (2020). Defining compassion in a hospital setting: Consensus on the characteristics that comprise compassion from researchers in the field. *Contemporary Nurse, 56*(2), 146–159. 10.1080/10376178.2020.1759437

Fairburn, Christopher G., & Cooper, Zafra (2011). Therapist competence, therapy quality, and therapist training. *Behaviour Research and Therapy*, 49, 373–378. 10.1016/j.brat.2011.03.005.

Handel, M. J. (2003). Skills mismatch in the labor market. *Annual Review of Sociology, 29*, 135–165.

Heinze, K., Suwanabol, P. A., Vitous, C. A., Abrahamse, P., Gibson, K., Lansing, B., & Mody, L. (2020). A Survey of Patient Perspectives on Approach to Health Care: Focus on Physician Competency and Compassion. *Journal of Patient Experience*, 1044–1053. 10.1177/2374373520968447

Hogston, R., & Marjoram, B. (2007). *Foundations of nursing practice: leading the way.* Palgrave.

Langins, M., & Borgermans, L. (2016). Strengthening a competent health workforce for the provision of coordinated/integrated health services. *International Journal of Integrated Care (IJIC), 16*(6).

Lee, Y., & Seomun, G. (2016). Compassion competence in nurses. *Advances in Nursing Science, 39*(2), E54–E66.

Liddell, A. E., Allan, S., & Goss, K. (2017). Therapist competencies necessary for the delivery of compassion-focused therapy: A Delphi study. *Psychology and Psychotherapy: Theory, Research and Practice, 90*(2), 156–176. 10.1111/papt.12105

Lown, B. A., Rosen, J., & Marttila, J. (2011). An agenda for improving compassionate care: a survey shows about half of patients say such care is missing. *Health Affairs, 30,* 1772–1778.

Ortega-Galán, Á. M., Ruiz-Fernández, M. D., Carmona-Rega, M. I., Cabrera-Troya, J., Ortíz-Amo, R., & Ibáñez-Masero, O. (2019). Competence and Compassion: Key Elements of Professional Care at the End of Life From Caregiver's Perspective. *American Journal of Hospice and Palliative Medicine®, 36*(6), 485–491. 10.1177/1049909118816662

Sharp, S., McAllister, M., & Broadbent, M. (2016). The vital blend of clinical competence and compassion: How patients experience person-centred care. *Contemporary Nurse, 52*(2–3), 300–312. 10.1080/10376178.2015.1020981

Sharpless, B. A., & Barber, J. P. (2009). A conceptual and empirical review of the meaning, measurement, development, and teaching of intervention competence in clinical psychology. *Clinical Psychology Review, 29*(1), 47–56. 10.1016/j.cpr.2008.09.008

Tehranineshat, B., Rakhshan, M., Torabizadeh, C., & Fararouei, M. (2018). Nurses', patients', and family caregivers' perceptions of compassionate nursing care. *Nursing Ethics.* 10.1177/0969733018777884

# 13

# THE PRACTICE AND APPLICATIONS OF COMPASSION STRENGTHS

### TRY AND APPLY

In the final chapter you can draw on all the knowledge you have gained about each strength and explore ways to try them out before you apply them to your practice. You can look at how each strength both individually and combined can be used in a range of settings and for a multitude of purposes.

## Introduction

At this point, you will have learned about compassion, its history, perspectives on if it is an emotion, behaviour, or both, and things that hinder or enable compassion. You have measured yourself for strengths and should now know what your compassion strengths are. You have explored each of the strengths in detail and how you can apply them to your work. Now, we have arrived at the Try and Apply section of the META model, where with these exercises all the strengths you have learned can be applied to your practice. In this chapter you will learn:

1. How to develop and apply compassion strengths for individuals
2. How to build compassionate organisations using strengths
3. How to apply strengths to different situations with clients and patients
4. How strengths can be used with positive psychology

## Compassion strengths for individuals

Now that you have explored all the different compassion strengths, the indicators and types that go with them, it can help to first start with an intention for how you will go forward with this information and apply it to your practice.

DOI: 10.4324/9781003276425-13

My compassion strengths intention:

_____

_____

_____

_____

_____

## The REPS method

To help with your intention and development of compassion strengths you can use the REPS methods. If we think of strengths as the muscles behind our compassion, just like when we work out in the gym, we can lose our compassion strengths if we stop exercising them. To keep and strengthen our compassion, we must cultivate and work on our compassion strengths regularly. Inspired by exercise and the idea that compassion is a strength, I devised the **REPS** method. **REPS** is a simple acronym for **Reflection, Example, Practice, Strengthen**. Like a workout, you can focus on one specific strength, or do a full body compassion strength workout. The key thing to remember is that daily repetition leads to increased strength and compassionate conditioning.

## Reflect

A wonderful place to start is by asking yourself and reflecting on the compassion strengths you already use and what you would like to work on. This is a chance to be mindful. Use mindfulness if you wish. Think about how you use your strengths, is there another way you can implement the strength or strengths into practice? What strengths do you need to work on more so that you can become your best self in that area? Reflect on what gets in the way and what you can do to overcome this barrier.

What compassion strengths am I already using?

_____

_____

_____

_____

_____

In what situation have used a particular strength and how did it help?

_____

_____

_____

_____

_____

What compassion strength would I like to work on?

_____

_____

_____

_____

_____

What gets in the way of me using my strengths?

_____

_____

_____

_____

_____

What enables me to develop and practice my compassion strengths?

_____

_____

_____

_____

_____

## Example

What examples can you give to evidence the indicators of your compassion strengths?

**TABLE 13.1** Example of the indicators of your compassion strengths

| Compassion strength | Indicator | How you might express this in your practice |
| --- | --- | --- |
| Self-care | | |
| Character | | |
| Communication | | |
| Connection | | |
| Competence | | |
| Engagement | | |
| Interpersonal | | |
| Empathy | | |

## Practice

Use the table below to guide you and include the compassion strengths and the indicators that would help you develop your compassion. You can do these at your work and or at home with others not related to your professions such as family and friends. By developing your compassion strengths outside of work, you will become stronger at understating people which will transfer over into your clinical work.

**TABLE 13.2** Practice sheet for your compassion strengths

| Compassion strength and its indicators: (for example, self-care - exercise) |
|---|
| What barriers might I face? |
| What will I do to overcome them? |
| How will this help your compassionate practice? |
| What three things can you do right now?<br><br>1.<br>2.<br>3. |

## Strengthen

Here we are aiming to strengthen each and our overall compassion strengths. We want to achieve the right amount of strength, the "just right" where we are using the right amount of this strength. Jot down and reflect on your answer for how you think your compassion strengths might look when being used. You can do this for an individual strength or them all. This will help you strengthen your awareness and your compassion strengths.

## The right amount of compassion strength

Is it possible for someone to have too much compassion, and suffer as a result? Of course, if they are putting themselves in the way of suffering, they can experience burnout and empathy/compassion fatigue. They can also be motivated to do too much and risk their safety or lives for others. For example, driving too fast to get to someone in need and risking causing more harm and suffering by creating an accident on the road.

Equally, we want to be using the "right amount" when demonstrating our strengths but for whatever reason, whether that be because we are stressed, or do not have the training at that time, we just cannot seem to demonstrate each strength in the way we would like. It can therefore help to think of our strengths as being on a continuum, where just like a physical strength we might use it too much, or too little, and maybe external things prevent us from expressing our compassion strengths in the ways that we'd like. We want to find the right amount of strength to use, both on ourselves and others. What do our strengths look like at each end of the continuum and what is the right amount we are aiming for?

Consider someone who uses too much communication. They might talk over the patient or talk too much and not listen to others. Someone who uses too little communication might not speak at all and come across as uninterested in the client. Becoming aware of our compassion strengths and what they look like at each end of the spectrum can help us become more proficient with them in practice. Some refer to this as the Golden mean (Niemiec, 2017). The golden mean was first talked about by Aristotle in 400 BC and has been used to describe the balance between virtues.

**TABLE 13.3** The right amount of compassion strengths table

| Compassion strength | Too little | The right amount | Too much |
| --- | --- | --- | --- |
| Communication | Not responsive, quiet, blank expression | Active listening, Open body language, speaking clear | Talk too much, do not listen, closed body language |
| Empathy | Apathy, uncaring, cruel, not understanding others | Understanding, responding | Over-emotional attachment leads to burnout. |

*(Continued)*

**TABLE 13.3** (Continued)

| Compassion strength | Too little | The right amount | Too much |
|---|---|---|---|
| Character | Dismissive, cold, rude, cruel | Kindness, warmth, honesty, respect, appropriate humour, | Overly caring making patient feel uncomfortable |
| Connection | Distant, lack of interest in patient | Connecting to the other on a meaningful and professional level | Overly intense interest, which makes patient/ client feel uncomfortable |
| Interpersonal | Inability to communicate in a non-clinical way, non-team player | Ability to communicate with a wide range of people from diverse backgrounds and use appropriate language and speech | Overly flexible, or relying on a team to do your work |
| Self-care | Not looking after self, especially when it is needed. | Employs strategies into practice that benefit self and others' wellbeing | Hyper focused on self-care, doing so much to the point of exhaustion |
| Engagement | Not doing anything, below standard care | Going above normal duties to provide personalised care | Doing too much without considering the patient's need |
| Competence | Lacking the clinical skills required for your role | Using clinical skills in ways that are perceived as helping with compassion | Being too clinical or only relying upon these skills |
| Overall | Lacking compassion or kindness. Being hostile to others | Using the right balance of strengths appropriate for the situation | Too much compassion. Doing more than is necessary. Allowing your good nature to be taken advantage of |

What might my strength/s look like when it is being used properly?

_____
_____
_____
_____
_____

What would too much be like?

_____
_____
_____
_____
_____

What would too little be like?

_____
_____
_____
_____
_____

How could you bring balance back to this strength?

_____
_____
_____
_____
_____

How might too little, too much, or just the right amount affects you and your practice?

_____
_____
_____
_____
_____

## My compassion strengths diary

There is a good quote that I love that helps motivate me towards my goals and can do the same for you. It is, "not much adds up". This might not make sense but if you read it again and think about it, it is a great reminder that doing something even if it is a little bit, adds up over time. So, think about it this way, "not much adds up, especially if we do it every day. A wonderful way to strengthen your compassion strengths is to make a diary of your activities each week. Over time you will notice what you have done and how it has gone.

**TABLE 13.4** Compassion strengths diary log

| Day/time/ place | What was I doing | What compassion strengths did I use | How did I use them? | Thoughts, feelings, barriers, feedback? |
|---|---|---|---|---|
| Day: *Tues* Time: *11 am* Place: *work* | *In session with a client* | *Empathy Communication* | *Listening to understand the context of their situation* | *It helped me connect to my client on a deeper level* |
| Day Time Place | | | | |
| Day Time Place | | | | |
| Day Time Place | | | | |
| Day Time Place | | | | |
| Day Time Place | | | | |
| Day Time Place | | | | |

Keeping a diary of your progress is an evidenced way of ensuring that you will continue to develop and build your strengths. Make a note when you use a particular strength and how it affects those around you, including yourself. Taking note of what happened and how we responded with compassion can help us become aware of when we are making best use of this strength and under what conditions. You can track your progress and achievements. You can take note of what worked and when.

## My compassion when I am stressed and burned out

Now consider what you would be like if you were stressed, burned out, and feeling weighed down by the pressure of your work. What would you be like? How compassionate would you be?

_____

_____

_____

_____

_____

Now consider what you would do to address this and the self-care activities you would use to reduce these feelings and improve your wellbeing.

_____

_____

_____

_____

_____

## Self-care emergency

In an emergency, it is helpful to think of activities we can put in place to counteract the impact of the event leading to further stress and pressure on our mental health and wellbeing. Something quick and easy activity such as taking a 1-minute mindful moment or grounding exercise to recentre yourself can make a massive difference for your ability to continue without the burden of care becomes too much.

With self-care, there is evidence that this also benefits healthcare practitioners when they know what they want to do, why they need it, and simple steps to achieve their goals. It follows a When-Then plan to help you develop the positive habits that will help you build your compassion strengths. For example, if you can identify what your triggers are, and your warning signs, then you can map this with an activity that helps you feel better. For example, tell yourself that when you feel (trigger) stressed at work Then you will go for a run after (self-care activity).

**TABLE 13.5** Self-care emergency log

| Event | Triggers/Warning signs | Feeling | Activity (hi/lo) |
|-------|------------------------|---------|------------------|
|       |                        |         |                  |
|       |                        |         |                  |
|       |                        |         |                  |
|       |                        |         |                  |
|       |                        |         |                  |
|       |                        |         |                  |

# Linking compassion strengths to wellbeing (PERMA)

Positive psychological well-being in the workplace can be achieved through finding meaning at work and being able to demonstrate competency in our abilities (Deci & Ryan, 2008). Well-being is significantly affected by negative personal and working conditions. At the same time when they are both positive, well-being flourishes and thus so does compassion. Cultivating compassionate healthcare cultures can help foster positive well-being and collective compassion raising awareness of the benefits of self-compassion and compassion for others (Vogus & McClelland, 2020).

A model of wellbeing that enables human flourishing is the PERMA model by Professor Marty Seligman. It consists of five key areas that lead to flourishing and positive wellbeing. They are Positive emotions, Engagement, Relationships (Positive), Meaning, and Accomplishment. There are techniques for learning how to develop in each area.

## Positive emotion

This is concerned with the things that make you feel good. When we are stressed, our negative biases come online, and we tend to see things as bad. However, we can counteract this by focusing on the positives. In doing so we become more optimistic. The broaden and build theory suggests that when we do this, we open ourselves up to more opportunities to gain experience and find ways to move forward.

## Engagement

Engagement in PERMA is different from compassion strength engagement. While engagement for PERMA means flow and fully attending to a task with complete focus, for compassion strengths it is about attending fully to the patient, doing the little things, and going above and beyond for others. This type of engagement relates to being engrossed in an activity to the point we lose track of time and find it rewarding. Examples are, playing an instrument, solving a puzzle, painting, or mediation.

## Relationships

This is about the relationships you have with people and the joy they bring to your life and boost your wellbeing. Connecting to people can give us a greater sense of meaning in our lives and help us foster strong friendships and bonds with those around us. Knowing and having someone who will be there for us when we experience bad days can help bring us back up again.

## Meaning

What is meaningful to you? This part of PERMA is about the things in life that have a deeper purpose that transcends beyond the self. Doing for others, kindness, volunteering, and donating to charity are great ways to express meaning. Being part of a spiritual group or church are ways that enable us to create a meaningful life.

## Accomplishment

Accomplishment is concerned with our goals and aspirations, the things we want to achieve that will help bolster our wellbeing. It is about becoming competent with the self in developing new skills. This does not just mean being competent at work, but in any area of life, and it is pursued for its own sake, regardless of the outcome.

The self-care strength includes physical, emotional, spiritual, social, professional, and psychological needs. PERMA has positive emotions, engagement, relationships, meaning, and accomplishment. Addressing our self-care needs places us in a state of optimal wellbeing and flourishing. This leads to happiness and more compassion for self and others.

What self-care/compassion strength activities can you link to PERMA?

_____
_____
_____
_____
_____

How do you feel when you experience these things?

_____
_____
_____
_____
_____

## Above point zero

For years, psychology (clinical) has been concerned with understanding and finding solutions to the various problems people face. However, recent developments and the advent of positive psychology have seen clinical terms such as dysfunction, illness, and problems, balanced with resilience, flourishing, and compassion (Gillham & Seligman, 1999; Seligman & Csikszentmihalyi, 2000). Rather than deal with what is wrong with a person, positive psychology looks at what is right with them. Positive psychology also asks what we can do after we help a patient overcome their suffering. The absence of suffering does not equate to a healthy life. It is often referred to as the zero point when a client has rid themselves of their woes, troubles, or suffering. However, in certain cases, patients report feeling that they have been left empty (Seligman, 2007). When the tank gets empty, we need to fill it with things that nourish us and help us flourish.

While it would be ideal for us to lift others and ourselves above suffering to a place of continuous positive experience, as life is tough it is not realistic to think this way. A more holistic perspective considers the two both suffering and positive experiences to be at either end of the spectrum of human experience that interacts at different time points. Not only does compassion keeps us connected to each other, but our experiences both good and bad. It helps us recognise when we and others are in need and when those needs have been addressed.

The aim of any healthcare organisation and the people who work within it is to alleviate suffering. The ideal path is to move from suffering to non-suffering. In taking this further, positive psychology encourages us to think about what happens after we reduce suffering, what the patient can do, or what can we do to support them towards improving their wellbeing after we have helped the reduction of suffering. This can be referred to as point zero, as in no-suffering, and is based upon the idea that the absence of illness or distress does not necessarily equate to healthy living. At the same time, if our patient is not suffering, we are more likely to not need to provide compassion, but at the same time, we can still try to at least improve their wellbeing. Equally, we should think about how we can rise above our situation once we have arrived at a place of non-suffering and take them and us above point zero. Just like suffering and the reduction of it, moving above the zero point usually follows a non-linear process. Life is not easy and there will always be suffering from things that will bring us down from a place of well-being and require a compassionate and positive response from self to other and self to self.

## Taking others above point zero

The aim of this exercise is not only to get you to think about and raise your awareness of suffering but to consider what you can do to alleviate it and take the person above suffering. With the help of the compassion strengths and each exercise, you should be able to build on this and develop your abilities further.

What do your patients/clients/service users suffer with?

_____

_____

_____

_____

_____

What can you do to reduce that suffering?

_____

_____

_____
_____
_____

How can you help them move above suffering, what is it that they need?

_____
_____
_____
_____
_____

What can you teach them to improve their physical and mental well-being and avoid further suffering?

_____
_____
_____
_____
_____

What strengths will you use?

_____
_____
_____
_____
_____

Understanding what the people we care for are suffering from, what it looks like when that suffering has gone, and what we can do to improve their well-being, are the first important steps to becoming a compassionate practitioner. Next, we need to understand what the strengths are that help us to recognise suffering, alleviate it, and help move others to a place of wellbeing and flourishing. We can achieve the reduction of suffering using each strength. This, in turn, can also take us above zero where both the patients and our well-being, joy, and happiness are increased because of giving and receiving compassion.

## How are you using compassion strengths with others?

How can you use your compassion strengths to alleviate suffering and take others above the zero point? For example, empathy helps us recognise the needs and suffering of others. Using aspects of our compassionate character, communication, and interpersonal skills we communicate our understanding without judgement and show warmth, while listening helps us connect to the person on a deeper level to their anguish. This helps us engage in actions that alleviate their suffering using our clinical competence to achieve this.

**TABLE 13.6** Using compassion strengths to take others above point zero

| Strength | How are you using it on others? | What are the potential outcomes of this? (PERMA) |
|---|---|---|
| Character | | |
| Empathy | | |
| Interpersonal | | |
| Communication | | |
| Connection | | |
| Engagement | | |
| Competence | | |
| Self-care | | |

## What compassion strengths are you using for yourself?

The remarkable thing about compassion strengths is that they can be turned inward. For example, you might be cursing yourself for a mistake you have made, but rather than treat yourself badly, you could use your strengths in various helpful ways. The character of being non-judgemental, to not judge yourself harshly. Empathy to empathise with your situation or the painful parts of the self that are hurting. Interpersonal skills and communication to speak with the different parts of self that are competing with one another with compassion. Connection to connect to the part of you that is wounded as a result of your mistake. Engagement to attend to the little things you can do for yourself in that situation and self-care strategies such as self-compassion to soothe yourself, and your competence to know what clinical skills can support you. Integrate them into yourself and become strong and compassionate. How can you use your compassion strengths to take yourself above the zero point? (See Table 13.7.)

## Daily compassion exercise

Pick a compassion strength and think about how you can use it that day either on yourself or others. The next day chose another, and then another, and continue to do this each day. Build up a weekly exercise regime where you work on a different strength each day.

## My compassionate day imagery exercise

Imagine your perfect compassionate day in which you use all your strengths to the best of your abilities. Think about and see what kind of impact they have on your

**TABLE 13.7** Using your compassion strengths to take you above point zero

| Strength | How are you using it on yourself? | What are the potential outcomes of this? (PERMA) |
|---|---|---|
| Character | | |
| Empathy | | |
| Interpersonal | | |
| Communication | | |
| Connection | | |
| Engagement | | |
| Competence | | |
| Self-care | | |

patients, their family, and your colleagues. Bring into awareness all the movements, feelings, and compassionate behaviours that you see yourself doing. Make them as vivid as you can. What will you be doing, which strengths are you using and how? Who are you with, and how are they reacting to you using your compassion strengths? Do not worry if you cannot. You can always write this down in your journal.

_____

_____

_____

_____

_____

## The end of my compassionate day

A simple exercise you can do is at the end of each day, try to write down all the compassionate things that you did and what strengths you used. Aim for a minimum of three but do not stop there if there are more.

1. _____
2. _____
3. _____
4. _____
5. _____
6. _____

## What a compassionate practitioner looks like now

Remember in the second chapter when you were asked to draw what a compassionate practitioner looked like? Now that you had read the book and gone through each exercise, has anything changed? Repeat the exercise then compare this drawing/description with the earlier one you did.

---

### BOX 13.1 WHAT A COMPASSIONATE PRACTITIONER LOOKS LIKE NOW

---

In addition to this, take the compassion strengths questionnaire to see if there are any changes in your scores from when you completed it the first time round.

## Developing compassion strengths with others/colleagues

In this section, we will focus on what you can do to bring compassion strengths into your workplace with colleagues. Compassion strengths can be practiced for both self and others. This can be helpful to you and the people you work with, whether they be colleagues or clients. Working with strengths in this way creates a more holistic view of compassion.

## Mirroring a compassion strength role model

Role modelling is a terrific way to develop your compassion. For this exercise, look for people who embody the compassion strengths in this book and use them effectively in their work.

What is it about this person that makes them a key role model for compassion strengths?

_____

_____

_____

_____

_____

How can you incorporate what they do into your practice?

_____

_____

_____

_____

_____

## Compassion strengths and the definition of compassion

The accepted definition of compassion is to be aware of another's suffering, with the motivation and action to alleviate it. Here I will show how compassion strengths achieve each aspect of the definition.

### Awareness of suffering

The first step involves being aware of another's suffering. To do this the compassion strengths of connection, character, communication, and interpersonal skills can be used. Becoming aware of another's suffering requires the compassionate character of courage to be present with distress, which then leads to the motivation to act upon it.

### Motivation to act

For the next step, you must be motivated to act upon that suffering. To achieve this, empathy can give us insight into another's situation, while self-care techniques help us manage our distress tolerance so that we feel comfortable moving toward the suffering.

### Actions to relive suffering

In the last step, you can draw on compassion strengths of character, engagement, and competence to provide kindness, encouragement, or another compassionate characteristic, engage with their needs and use clinical competence to treat them and facilitate change.

### What strengths work best together in your work with others?

Whose compassion strengths do you admire, and what is it about them that you like most?

_____

_____

_____

_____

_____

Think about which strengths you use together and what works best in what situation

_____

_____

_____

_____

_____

Think about the impact your compassion strengths and how you perform as a practitioner have on you and those around you. There might be ones that you use most that will affect how you care for others differently.

_____

_____

_____

_____

_____

How often when you demonstrate these strengths, including the strongest ones you use most, and do they lead to improved performance.

_____

_____

_____

_____

_____

How do you feel when using these strengths? Using your compassion strengths often, and with a greater impact on self and others, will add to the good feelings that come from improved performance and acts of compassion that make a real difference to your work. With your strength's builder, you can check and assess your progress throughout each of the exercises and strengths.

_____

_____

_____

_____

_____

## Applications of compassion strengths in learning and practice

In this section, we will turn to the applications of compassion strengths in various situations and organisational levels. We will cover how to develop compassionate individuals, teams, leaders, managers, and organisations. It will also provide examples of how compassion strengths can be used in many different scenarios involving patients or clients. But first, let us explore how compassion strengths can help you support the people you care for and take them above the zero point.

## How compassion strengths can help improve compassionate practice and the practitioner

To be compassionate means to be aware of clients' and patients suffering, be emotionally responsive to this, and address the needs of others. It also means to be self-aware and treat yourself with compassion. This section will now apply compassion strengths to a series of principles in healthcare, showing how they can be used in training and practice.

## Improve awareness of patients' needs and suffering

To improve awareness of patients and their suffering, practitioners need to use empathy, character, and connection to be non-judgemental, sympathetic, and understanding of these needs. This can be helped by using engagement to spend time with patients and take their perspectives. Learn about them and wonder what happened for them to end up in your care.

## Improve self-awareness and self-compassion

Improving your self-awareness can help you manage tricky situations and dis-tressing feelings. Things you can do is use self-care, reflection, mindfulness, and personal pursuits that build wellbeing. Having a support network and connection to others build you too. Observing how you feel and being non-judgmental of your feelings and treating yourself with self-compassion and kindness helps build compassion strengths. Do things that help you decompress, go for a walk, or take a less stressful route home even if it is longer.

## Treat others/colleagues with compassion

Use empathy, the character of kindness, and non-judgement to consider your colleague's perspective. Prepare in advance before meetings and interactions. Treat your time together with respect and support them where you can.

## How compassion strengths can improve practice and education at the organisational level

### Candidate selection

Use compassion strength material as training and recruitment exercises to identify individuals with the capacity to be compassionate. Building on the vignettes, organisations can bring them into the interview process and ask candidates to reflect on them while recruiters look out for compassion strengths.

## Training staff to demonstrate compassionate strengths

Courses can be developed using the compassion strengths model as the foundation for compassion in your practice. The worksheets in this chapter can be used and adapted to fit your profession.

## Assessment

The BCSI can be used to assess practitioners for compassion strengths in the workplace. This can be done as a self-assessment exercise, assessment from educators and managers, or patients to assess their practitioner's compassion.

## For curriculum

Assessment in the workplace using the compassion strength indicators and assessment tools. The education exercises will support students learning about compassion with activities that encourage the development of compassion strengths. They can be tailored to suit your practice and people at each stage of their profession.

## For leaders and managers

Develop your compassion strengths and show them to staff. Incorporate the compassion strengths into your workplace to promote them and create a sense of compassion through your staff and organisation. Staff members are more likely to respond with compassion when they are treated with compassion and given the platforms to enable it to grow and show. Create compassion rewards and celebrate these achievements in the same way you might do the same with targets. Give staff the space to talk openly about their feelings, and what affects their mental health and wellbeing, and provide opportunities for them to develop self-care.

## A compassion strength perspective approach for collaborating with different clients and patients

Quite often we meet a wide range of patients and clients that can be categorised as being needy, demanding, dependant, manipulative, or even self-destructive. Nomenclature such as this does not lend itself to compassion. Indeed, people will demonstrate behaviours that practitioners will find frustrating. However, behind every behaviour, there is a reason or multitude of reasons to explain why they are that way which is not clear on the surface. Therefore, strong compassionate understanding is needed so that pain can be heard and people cared for.

Using examples of each patient, let us look at them through the lens of compassion and see how the compassion strengths approach can help shift the perspective.

## Dependent patients/clients

While on the surface, they may seem dependent, these patients are annoyed and uncomfortable with the idea of being deserted. Hence, they demand more personal time from the practitioner. Thus, it is essential to maintain a professional demeanour with well-established boundaries. It can help to involve the patient in decision-making. Using your compassion strengths, assure them that they will not be abandoned/neglected and will be given full attention in later visits also.

## Demanding patients/clients

Patients considered demanding can often be aggressive and intimidating and do not want to go through each step of assessments or treatment. In such a situation the practitioner can apply character and empathy to avoid judgement and empathetically ensure the patient that they will get the care they need and there is no need to show anger.

## Manipulative patients/clients

Clients who have been rejected previously often revisit the practitioner in cycles of help-seeking/rejecting treatment and do not improve despite proper advice. Their firm belief that their health cannot improve even puts the healthcare professionals in doubt about what they can do to treat them. However, the practitioner in such circumstances should use empathy and communication to understand and listen to their problems attentively while sharing frustration over poor outcomes. The practitioner must reformulate the treatment plan with the patient after having set limitations over expectations.

## Self-destructive patients/clients

Patients with underlying anxiety or depression are often hopeless about their condition and fear failure. Their problems persist despite adequate counselling and management. The patient continues self-destructive habits, and the healthcare professional considers themselves ineffective and responsible for their patient's lack of progress. The practitioner must use empathy, connection, and active listening to prioritise the patient's immediate concerns and expectations. They can help explore reasons for non-adherence to therapy and offer alternative solutions. They must identify all the contributing factors and approach the patient with a non-judgemental and caring character. Using interpersonal skills, you can involve the patient by asking them about the possible cause of poor outcomes and potential solutions that would foster a more collaborative relationship leading to therapeutic success.

Empathy is a key strength of compassion that can be used to understand the experiences of clients who behave in this way. What other strengths might you use in such situations? Think about how you can combine strengths to show compassion.

Questions to ask yourself when with patients or colleagues are to avoid judgement and look beyond the presenting behaviours.

What can I do for this person?

_____
_____
_____
_____
_____

How would I feel if I were in this person's position?

_____
_____
_____
_____
_____

How does this person's story make me feel?

_____
_____
_____
_____
_____

What does this person need from me?

_____
_____
_____
_____
_____

What strengths can I use to help this person?

_____
_____
_____
_____
_____

## *Using compassion strengths when breaking difficult news*

Imagine the following scenario. You have just been given a life-changing diagnosis and the practitioner tells you raw facts about your condition and horrible truths in such a way that you feel worse about the delivery of the news than the news itself. Breaking unwelcome news that is potentially devastating to a person's life, needs to be approached with sensitivity and understanding of their expectations.

When breaking unwelcome news, compassionate empathic communication is required. This can help when dealing with the patient's reaction. Without these skills, there is a risk of making the relationship between patient and practitioner worse and their hope of supporting them through this. Compassion strengths such as communication, interpersonal skills, empathy, and connection can assist the practitioner in the following ways:

Before the meeting, it is helpful to prepare how you will deliver the news, and what you will do in response to their reaction. Compassionate communication such as sitting open and relaxed, and using eye contact in a private place away from others can help. Open-ended questions can help get a feel for the patient's knowledge and awareness of their condition and how prepared they are for the news. Explore how much information they might want from you and in how much detail. This can take the pressure off knowing how much to tell them.

Empathy is key to assessing and providing the right emotional support in response to their reactions to hearing the bad news. This may range from anger, and denial, to disbelief and crying. Nevertheless, the practitioner must validate their feelings, move close and provide comfort to them, hold their hand, and express their disappointment. Give them quiet moments to process the news before asking further questions. Interpersonal skills can be used to involve the patient in their care plan. While connection and engagement might be used to go the extra mile for them.

## Conclusion

We have come to the end of this book. I hope that you have enjoyed reading it but most of all, I hope that you have learned a lot about your compassion strengths. As you go forward with the things you have learned I encourage you to continue putting into practice the skills and indicators of each strength so that you can become your strongest compassionate self, and that what you do helps you and others to flourish. I wish you all the absolute best in your progress as you continue to build and maintain your compassion strengths and apply them to your own life and practice.

What do I know now that I did not before?

_____

_____

_____

_____

_____

# References

Deci, Edward L., & Ryan, Richard M. (2008). Facilitating optimal motivation and psychological well-being across life's domains. Canadian Psychology/Psychologie canadienne, 49, 14–23. 10.1037/0708-5591.49.1.14

Gillham, J. E., & Seligman, M. E. (1999). Footsteps on the road to a positive psychology. *Behaviour Research and Therapy, 37*(1), S163–S173. 10.1016/S0005-7967(99)00055-8

Niemiec, R. M. (2017). *Character strengths interventions: A field guide for practitioners.* Hogrefe Publishing.

Seligman, M. E. (2007). *Learned Optimism: How to Change Your Mind and Your Life* (3rd ed.): Vintage Books.

Seligman, M. E., & Csikszentmihalyi, M. (2000). Positive psychology: An introduction. *American Psychologist, 55*(1), 5–14. DOI: 10.1037//0003-066X.55.1.5

Vogus, T. J., & McClelland, L. E. (2020). Actions, style and practices: how leaders ensure compassionate care delivery. *BMJ Leader, 4*(2). 10.1136/leader-2020-000235

# INDEX

Note: Locators in *italic* and **bold** refer to figures and tables, respectively.

Printed in the United States
by Baker & Taylor Publisher Services